Through the Eyes
of a Mother

Through the Eyes of a Mother

Harmful Assumptions

alina yates

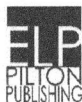

ELP
PILTON
PUBLISHING

ALINA BOOKS are published by

EL Pilton Publishing Co., Plano, Texas 75025

www.alinabooks.com
www.piltonpublishing.com

Some names, characters, businesses, organizations, and places have been
changed or altered to protect the identity of those individuals or places; and
any reference made to any individuals, places, organizations, and incidents
are merely from the narrator's point of view. The information in this
publication is generally consistent with those diagnosed with Severe
Hemophilia Type A, but none of the suggested care instructions or "End
Notes" are the opinion of any doctor, nurse, or hospital listed under the
Helpful Resources page. The author, publisher, or narrator is not responsible
for any of the information presented from other sources and cannot ensure
the efficiency or effectiveness of any product, service, or care indicated in
this book. Please consult your physician or a health care professional before
undertaking any medication or treatment programs stated in this
publication.

For more information on Alina Books, visit, **www.alinabooks.com** for up-to-
date information on the authors or to place an order.

Library of Congress Cataloging-in-Publication Data

Alina Yates.
        Through the Eyes of a Mother / by Alina Yates.

ISBN 978-0-9887933-0-9

Printed in the United States of America
Cover design by Angel A. Allen

for Eric and Jaden

CONTENTS

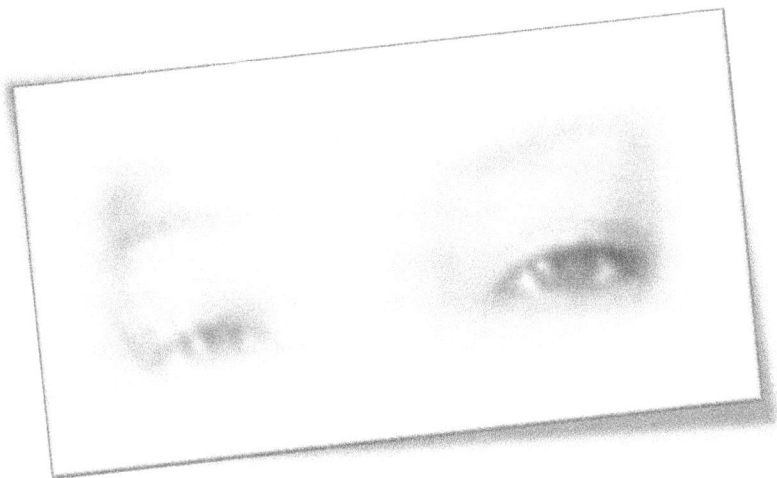

THE SHOCK WAVE

NOVEMBER 1997

"It doesn't matter what the doctors, specialist, or nurses say in regards to the care of my child, I just wanted them to *see* and *appreciate* my point of view—

Through the Eyes of a Mother!"

—*Gamila*

Introduction

DO YOU HAVE:
frequent nose bleeds
heavy menstrual bleeding
periods longer than seven days
excessive gum bleeding
bleeding after minor injuries
a migraine diagnosis?

If you answered yes to any of these, you could have a bleeding disorder such as **von Willebrand Disease (VWD)** or **Hemophilia**. Von Willebrand Disease is the most common bleeding disorder. According to the Centers for Disease Control—www.cdc.gov—VWD occurs with equal frequency in women and men, but women are more likely to experience symptoms. Of the women diagnosed with VWD, 95% reported heavy menstrual bleeding, 92% reported bleeding after minor injuries, and 76% reported excessive gum bleeding.

Hemophilia is a rare bleeding disorder that occurs primarily in boys. According to the Hemophilia Federation of America,[1] approximately 400 babies a year are born with hemophilia. Hemophilia A is the most severe and it is four times more common than Hemophilia B. Of the more than 400,000 people living across the globe with the disorder, about 20,000 are in the U.S.

[1] HFA - http://www.hemophiliafed.org/bleeding-disorders/hemophilia/

Chapter One

A Rarity

CRISP, COLD breeze ruffled the gentle snowfall on November 15, 1997. It was a bitter 32 degrees and the season had just begun. That first layer of snow was thin, but it was a subtle indication of what was to come that winter in Detroit. But even as the frosty weather began, a warm feeling seemed to swaddle the air like a quilt. By November 27th the temperature had risen to 39 degrees and the fragile layer of snow had melted away.

The new mother exhibited a hint of exhaustion as she made the lengthy walk across the hospital parking lot. Dad walked behind her, patiently guiding her toward the doors. As the couple entered the hospital, their breath trailed visibly behind them like vapor.

The new mother had been released several days earlier—without her baby boy. Baby Chris was yellow when he was born, and he had respiratory problems. The doctors said he had jaundice and it was standard procedure to keep him in until they were certain that his liver was functioning normally. The new mother visited her baby all day every day. It wasn't long before she realized that there was nothing normal about his hospital stay.

With baby steps and slow movements, Gamila finally made it to the Nursery Care Unit on the fourth floor. From the door of the unit she could see Chris's breathing tubes, the leads from his cardiac monitor, and the incubator hood that protected his small body. But Chris didn't look right. He was lying motionless on his back, and it seemed as though there were more tubes than she remembered.

Gamila washed her hands and robed for the visit. As she moved closer, a perplexed expression came over her face. Chris wasn't his usual jolly self. He looked flaccid, pale, and listless. It seemed as if the life had been sucked right out of him.

"What's going on here?"

"What do you mean?" asked the nurse.

"What do you mean, 'what do you mean'?" said Gamila with a dismissive glance. As she tried to figure out what was different from the night before, her eyes followed the tubing that was connected to Chris. "Do you have him in a girl's diaper? Why is his diaper pink? Look, just give me a diaper so I can change him."

The nurse walked over to the new parents. She figured she would just change the diaper and get on with her shift. "We don't have pink diapers here. I'll change him." She slowly undid the adhesive strips on the baby's diaper. "It should be OK," she added softly. Her face said something entirely different.

Gamila's heart sank into the pit of her aching stomach. She was already slightly hunched over from the natural birth of baby Chris days earlier, and now her eyes were bulging.

"What the *hell* did you do to my baby?" Gamila snarled.

"Well . . . I don't know. It should be fine. Just . . . just . . . let me clean him up and change his diaper." The nurse's words were unhurried, cautious.

"Why is there a puddle of blood in my baby's diaper?" roared Gamila. "What the hell is going on in here? Get the damn doctor who did this RIGHT NOW!" Gamila stared in shock for a few moments at her helpless newborn before her motherly instincts went into overdrive. "Give me the diaper. I will clean my baby up and you just call the doctor who did this . . . NOW!" As she was cleaning Chris up, she noticed the nasty, amateur-looking sutures on him. "What are these stitches for and why do they look like this?"

"It's normal to have a little bleeding after circumcision," the nurse explained.

"Does this look like a *little* blood to you? And look at my baby, he's pale, limp, and blinking his eyes slowly like he's exhausted. He's lost too much blood. Don't you see that? You need to call the doctor who did this to my baby."

"Well, that doctor's not on duty."

"I don't care where he is. I want him here, NOW. He needs to explain what he did and why my son is bleeding profusely. And he needs to fix it, plain and simple."

"But ..." The nurse could practically see the steam pouring from Gamila's head. Rightfully so, she thought, but she had to try to calm the enraged mother. "He's at home with his family you know, and ..."

Gamila turned and looked the nurse in the eye. "I don't give a damn where he is or who he's with. You need to get him here. If he's not here within the hour I'm going to blame you for this."

"I'll. . . I'll call him right now," the nurse spluttered as she left the room.

The doctor arrived forty-five minutes later. Chris's diaper was blood-soaked again and he was even paler and more exhausted. Gamila could see that her baby was getting weaker.

"It's OK. It is normal for the baby to have some bleeding after a circumcision," the doctor insisted.

"Does that look like a *little blood* to you?" Gamila asked through gritted teeth. She remained calm, but she couldn't hide the fuming, disturbed expression on her face.

"It's going to be OK. Let me take a look." The doctor opened the diaper and an unmistakable look of surprise and puzzlement washed over him. He hesitated for a moment before offering a paltry explanation. "I didn't understand why he was bleeding so much after the procedure, but I thought it would subside." The doctor paused. "He should be OK."

"Look, I'm tired of both of you. If you don't fix him, then I will," said Gamila.

"OK. OK. Just give me a minute. I can fix it. I can fix it." The doctor was nervous.

Gamila was at breaking point. She felt that the doctor wasn't telling her the whole story, but time was a luxury she didn't have. She had to think. She had to focus on the doctor fixing her baby. She found herself thinking *for* the doctor.

"You need to remove this horrible stitch job you did and do it right. You also need to find out why there's so much blood. Do you know why?"

"I can fix it," the doctor repeated.

The new father had been standing by, watching in silence. He was stunned by what he'd seen. "I think I'm going to throw up," he muttered.

"You throw up and I'mma kick your butt," Gamila whispered.

Gamila was no one to be toyed with. The father glanced at her and knew she wasn't playing. The doctors had made the mistake of thinking that she was just another young mother they could manipulate and intimidate. They had no idea that Gamila was just as unique as her name. Once you felt her wrath—especially when it came to her children—you wouldn't make the same mistake again.

"OK," replied the father.

"OK, I can't do this while you are here." The doctor's accent was getting thicker by the minute.

"You're going to have to," Gamila stated matter-of-factly.

"I have to sterilize the area to do the procedure. You can't be here." A knot of nervousness and frustration lingered in the doctor's tight throat.

"Just do it *doctor*, or I will," Gamila ordered.

"You know how to do stitches?" the father whispered, leaning in close to Gamila.

"Shut up," Gamila hissed.

The doctor wasn't really paying attention to the baby's parents, but he was concerned to fix his mistake. He waved his hands in the air as if to surrender. "OK. OK. We have to sterilize the area and you two have to be sterile too."

The nurse sterilized the area as the doctor spread Chris's little arms and legs wide, strapping them down tight so he couldn't move. The child looked like Jesus on the cross as the doctor began the procedure.

It was horrific to watch. Gamila wanted to pass out. Her heart ached, her lungs could barely breathe, and it felt as if her soul was being ripped from her body.

"I'm gonna pass out," said the father.

"You pass out and I'mma kick your butt," Gamila whispered.

"OK," the father said. He was on the verge of tears.

Gamila's eyes were glued to the doctor. His hands were shaking at first like an anxious Ralph Furley— Don Knotts's character on *Three's Company*—but he soon began moving quickly and professionally. His nervousness dissipated and his stitching skills seemed to have been miraculously perfected.

However impressed Gamila was watching the doctor, she couldn't ignore Chris's chilling screams. Her heart was bleeding for her newborn son.

"I can't watch this," the father whispered. "I think I'mma be sick."

"We gotta stay alert. Pull it together," Gamila snapped. She wanted to turn away too, but her mother's instincts wouldn't allow it. This procedure had to be done right. The mistake had to be corrected. She didn't want the doctor to screw up again and she made herself watch every move he made.

The doctor finished and his stitches were perfect. The procedure had gone well, but blood was still oozing from Chris's penis.

"He's still bleeding." Gamila wanted to breakdown and cry.

"OK. Let's just give it some time to stop." The doctor looked confused. He knew he'd done the procedure correctly this time and he couldn't understand why the baby was still bleeding. "Let me run some tests."

Gamila didn't want to leave baby Chris, but she had to go home and rest.

* * *

The day Gamila was scheduled to pick up her baby from the hospital, she received a phone call. The doctor's tone was sharp and dry. He sounded troubled.

Gamila's heart plunged and she could've sworn she heard a hard thump in her chest. She was surprised that the doctor didn't hear it, or feel her hands trembling through the phone.

"We had to give the baby some plasma," the doctor finally told her. "A test confirmed that your son has a rare deficiency." The doctor paused, waiting for her response.

Gamila knew the doctor meant that her newborn had to have a blood transfusion, but she had no idea what he meant by a *rare deficiency*. She didn't respond.

"Your son has a factor VIII deficiency which prevents his blood from clotting normally. You will need to make an appointment with the hematologist at The Hospital, and they can tell you more."

The conversation was over. Gamila burst into tears. For the first time in her life she felt helpless. She didn't know her next move and she couldn't have been prepared for what was to come.

Chapter Two

In the Beginning
1997

Gamila's pain started with a muscle spasm. Her mom made an appointment for her at the trusted Wellness Clinic. Gamila had been going there since she was five and her mom was comfortable with the care they'd given her two daughters.

"It's sort of like a muscle spasm," Gamila told the doctor.

"Have you recently done anything that would cause it?"

"Not that I can think of. I run track, but I've been doing that for a while and I don't think. . ."

The doctor interrupted her. "Ah, that explains it then. It's just a muscle spasm causing cramps."

"I don't think so. This is no ordinary muscle spasm, and I think I would know if it was a muscle cramp, doctor. This is something different. The pain is different. It's constant."

The doctor wasn't interested in hearing any more. He barely examined her before making his assessment. "She'll be fine. Drink plenty of fluids," the doctor kept repeating.

Gamila tried to get an answer about why her pain was primarily in her lower back and on her right side. The doctor just told her that muscle spasms can occur in the abdomen and side.

"Oh, it will be OK. It's just muscle cramps. No need for this," said the doctor as he held up the small plastic cup containing Gamila's urine. He pressed his foot on the pedal of the trash can and dropped the sample inside.

Shock spread across Gamila's mother's face. Who does that? she thought. Gamila's mother was dumbfounded. She'd never seen a doctor throw out a sample like that before.

The doctor prescribed muscle relaxers and 800mg ibuprofen for Gamila's pain before sending them on their way.

Gamila was reluctant to take the muscle relaxers, but she'd taken ibuprofen before and she took that when she got home. The pain subsided within an hour. She was happy for the relief, but she knew that she wasn't just suffering from muscle cramps.

She decided to take one of the muscle relaxers that evening. It hit her hard and she didn't remember falling asleep. Gamila woke up on the sofa when she needed to go to the bathroom. Her pain returned as soon as she sat on the cold toilet seat. But now it was worse. It was so intense that she wanted to cry.

Gamila's mom took her back to the Wellness Clinic. Gamila was seen by a different doctor who diagnosed her with a kidney infection. The doctor prescribed antibiotics and gave Gamila more pain medication.

Gamila wasn't convinced that she had the right diagnosis, but she started taking the antibiotics anyway. She couldn't hold down any of the pills and she stopped taking them after the third day.

* * *

Months passed and Gamila was still in pain. She wasn't getting any better.

In the beginning, Gamila's mom had every intention of following the Wellness Clinic's doctors' orders. She trusted them. They'd provided good care to her daughters for years, but nothing was helping this time.

Gamila's mom wanted to take her daughter to another clinic, but the Wellness Clinic doctors were her primary care physicians. In other words, without a referral, Gamila couldn't step foot into another clinic or doctor's office unless her mom could pay for it out-of-pocket. Unfortunately, her mom couldn't afford to pay out-of-pocket to see a different doctor, and given the initial diagnosis of muscle spasms, there was no way that the Wellness Clinic would give Gamila a referral.

Gamila's mother had no choice but to take her daughter back to the Wellness Clinic. She made a third appointment.

When they got to the clinic Gamila tried pleading with the doctors. She explained that her pain was not due to muscle cramps or a kidney infection. She insisted that this pain was unlike anything she'd ever experienced, but the doctors refused to take her seriously.

They prescribed another medication and told Gamila she'd start feeling better once she started taking it. For the third time, Gamila was sent home with more pills and a new—but strangely similar—diagnosis.

By now, Gamila was in constant pain. She could keep the new medication down, but it certainly wasn't helping. In fact, Gamila felt the medication was making the pain worse, and she'd find out later that she was right. She'd had enough and she stopped taking all the pills.

* * *

Gamila had been making frequent torturous trips to the bathroom. She dreaded the cold, hard toilet seat because her pain seemed to intensify once she relaxed her bottom on that darn seat.

One night, Gamila's mother awoke to find Gamila on her hands and knees. She was crawling back to the sofa.

"What's wrong with you?" asked Gamila's mother.

"I'm in pain."

"You in that much pain where you can't walk?"

"Yeah!"

"This is ridiculous. I'm taking you to emergency."

The emergency room was typical of Detroit—everything happened at a snail's pace. If you weren't a heart patient, gunshot victim, stabbing victim (depending on where you were stabbed), an elderly person going into cardiac arrest, or brought in by an ambulance, you could forget about being seen in under four hours.

The chairs in the waiting room seemed designed for maximum discomfort. After more than five hours of sitting on the excruciatingly uncomfortable chairs, Gamila finally heard her name being called.

She noticed that there were very few actual examination *rooms* available. In fact, the emergency department was mostly made up of small spaces sectioned off by curtains. Gamila was relieved to get out of the waiting area, but she knew she'd still have to wait for at least another half hour before the doctor would push his way through the drawn curtain and examine her.

A nurse arrived first to get a brief medical history. She asked Gamila what she was in for and if she was currently taking any medications.

Gamila figured the best way not to increase her wait time was to start with the most severe symptoms and diagnosis. She told the nurse that she was in constant pain and that the doctors at the Wellness Clinic thought she had a kidney infection. Gamila didn't even bother mentioning the muscle spasm diagnosis. As Gamila began to explain that none of the medications she'd been prescribed had worked, the nurse cut her off.

"Did they do a pregnancy test?" The nurse looked down at Gamila's chart, scribbled something on it, looked up at Gamila, and asked again.

Gamila was perplexed. "Well, no, they didn't."

"That's what it sounds like to me, but we'll need to do a pregnancy test. It's the first test we perform. We'll also test for the kidney infection and anything else that may explain this pain you're experiencing."

The nurse's bedside manner was nothing to write home about, but Gamila was extremely relieved. Finally, after all these months, someone was listening to her—and taking steps to get to the root of the problem. Hearing the word "pregnant" was scary for Gamila, but it was an explanation that made sense. She'd never been pregnant, so it would explain why she'd never felt pain like this before.

After nine hours in the emergency room, Gamila and her mother finally had their answer. Gamila was pregnant.

Gamila's mother was understandably upset. She was upset that the doctors at the Wellness Clinic didn't do a pregnancy test, especially after so many appointments. She was also upset and concerned about the affect the pills could have on the baby.

* * *

Gamila's mom very reluctantly made another appointment at the Wellness Clinic. She would've taken her daughter anywhere else for prenatal care if she could've.

It was raining something fierce the day of Gamila's appointment, and her mom was ready to make her own brutal weather inside. Gamila's mother let the doctors know in no uncertain terms how furious she was that they'd repeatedly misdiagnosed her daughter.

Unsurprisingly, the doctors weren't too concerned. They immediately turned the situation around on Gamila and her mother.

"Well, she must've been hiding something from you Mom, because she should've known she was pregnant," one doctor insisted with a little smirk.

"How dare you! You're the doctor. I trusted *your* judgment." Gamila's mother was incredulous. "YOU should have known it was possible that she was pregnant. We came to you three times, *three times*, saw two different doctors, and neither of you thought to do a pregnancy test. The ER doctor insisted that should have been the first test you did. We're only back here now because you're her primary care physician."

"We can only follow the *symptoms*. Her *symptoms* pointed toward muscle spasms or a kidney infection." The doctor raised his voice. "Well, let's schedule an ultrasound to find out how far along she is and go from there. In the meantime, I'll prescribe some prenatal vitamins for your daughter."

It was clear that the doctor just wanted to end the conversation as quickly as possible. His demeanor said: just let it go and move on.

Gamila's mother got the sense that he was only concerned about justifying his actions, or, more precisely, his failure to act. She also got the sense that he didn't care that he'd screwed up. And she was right.

Until then, Gamila's body didn't show any visible signs that she was pregnant. She didn't have a tummy, her hips and thighs weren't swollen, her nose wasn't widened, nothing. The sickness and pain were the only hints her body gave her. But miraculously, a week after finding out that she was pregnant, Gamila's belly started to show. Her mom said the baby had been in hiding because it knew those idiots were trying to kill him.

The ultrasound revealed that Gamila was around seven months pregnant. No one could believe it and the doctors recommended another ultrasound. Gamila definitely thought they'd screwed up again.

In November, 1997 the arrival of baby boy Chris brought joy to the new mother and grandmother, but a darkness would soon overshadow their happiness.

Chapter Three

We've Overstayed Our Welcome

Gamila opened the back door of her Pontiac. As she strapped Chris into his car seat chaotic images of their last visit to the emergency room took shape in her mind. Chris looked at his mother playfully and gave a delightful baby giggle. He was slightly rocking his right leg, but the left one remained motionless.

Chris was only seven months, but Gamila had moved passed the "why me" stage by the time he was a month old. And by now, she'd also moved passed the weeping and angry stages. She'd never been one to cry much, but her life had had its moments when crying was her only possible release—like when the doctor first informed her of Chris's condition.

Some of the nurses and doctors at The Hospital would've suggested that Gamila hadn't moved passed her angry stage, but that was only because they interpreted her extreme caution, caring, and bluntness as anger. They expected her to act like an ordinary eighteen-year-old. They also thought they could manipulate her like an ordinary eighteen-year-old. What they failed to understand was that Gamila was a young mother whose child had a severe bleeding disorder. She had to grow up fast—faster than most young mothers.

Gamila pulled into the parking lot of The Hospital. She took a deep breath as she opened the back door of the car and unstrapped Chris.

"Hey, can you give me a hand here?" she shouted as she flagged down a security guard. She didn't really need his help, but it was around 2:00 a.m. and, as usual, the parking lot was pitch-black. As the security guard walked toward her, Gamila noticed that his sloppy, half-ironed clothes were hanging loosely off his frail body. This guy couldn't protect a fly, but he'll do. . . just so long as I don't have to walk through this dark parking lot by myself, she thought.

"Hey lady, I don't get paid for carrying luggage," he barked with a goofy smile.

"Yeah, I know you have better things to do... like arresting that pregnant lady for stealing a candy bar out of the vending machine."

"I see we have a comedian in the crowd," said the guard, smiling from ear to ear. He was actually excited to be doing more than just standing around pretending to be watching the entrance. In fact, he didn't really know what he was supposed to be protecting or preventing. All he knew was that being able to flirt with women was one of the few perks of his low-paying job.

"What crowd? Can you see a crowd? It's so damn dark out here I don't see how anyone can see anything."

"This is outside of my job duties," he playfully mentioned a second time.

"Can you just grab that bag in the front seat?" she said, running out of patience. "And watch what you're doing."

"OK, OK lady." He grabbed the bag from the front seat and followed her to the entrance of the emergency room.

The security guard didn't recognize Gamila until they were inside. Her reputation around the hospital had been duly noted by everyone, and looks of "here *she* comes" washed over most people's faces whenever they saw her. The guard recalled an encounter he'd had with her several months earlier. He'd learned his lesson the hard way. At first, he was offended by her coldness, her arrogance, but he eventually realized that anyone who was in and out of there so often would be frustrated. He also knew that she was there for only one reason—to get the care her son desperately needed.

"Can I help you?" snapped the receptionist as she chomped on a well-used piece of gum.

"Yes, my son Chris Malone has severe hemophilia A. We need to see a doctor for his treatment. . ."

The receptionist interrupted her. "What treatment? What is he being seen for?"

Gamila's nostrils flared. She counted to three in her head to avoid giving this receptionist or nurse or whatever she was a piece of her mind. Gamila took a slow, deep breath. "As I was saying, my son needs to see a doctor for treatment for a bleed in his knee. He has a knee bleed. . ."

The receptionist cut her off again. "His knee is bleeding?" She seemed extra agitated as she lifted her ample behind out of her chair and looked over the counter. "Is it bleeding *on the floor?* Do you need a towel or something?"

"OK. . . if you quit interrupting me, I can explain to you what the problem is so we can be on our way to the back. Jesus, this hospital really needs to get staff up here who aren't lazy, and someone who at least knows a little bit about medical care. Now, my son has hemophilia.[2] I'm sure you don't know what that is, so,

---

[2] Hemophilia is a rare disorder, also called factor VIII deficiency. It is caused by a mutated, missing, or defective factor VIII or clotting protein. A person with hemophilia has a problem with blood-clotting factors which are needed to stop bleeding after an injury. It is passed

to avoid the long-drawn-out interrogation that I typically have to go through every time I'm in this hospital, I thought I'd bypass all that and tell you that he needs to be treated. I have his medicine in my bag and I really don't have time to be wasting at this darn desk. Once you tell a *real nurse* that you have a patient out front who needs *immediate* medical attention, because he has a *knee bleed,* they'll send us to the back right away. Can you handle that?"

The woman was shocked to say the least. She was staring at Gamila who was glaring right back at her. Gamila wasn't going to budge until she had an answer. She gave the woman a few minutes before laying into her again.

"Hello? Can you call the emergency room doctor on duty so my son can get treated? He only has a small window here. If his treatment is not done *now*, he'll have to be admitted to the hospital." Gamila bent over and rubbed Chris's knee. It was getting hotter. She reached into her bag and pulled out an instant cold

---

down from the parents, but there are cases of spontaneous change in a gene. There are about 20,000 people in the U.S. with hemophilia. Hemophilia type A is the most severe. With severe hemophilia, bleeding episodes happen often, as frequently as once or twice a week. Most bleeds are spontaneous joint bleeds. For more information, see the *Helpful Resources* page. Source: www.acardocorp.org.

pack. She twisted the pack until she heard a pop and placed it on Chris's swollen knee.

The receptionist still hadn't called the doctor. She was watching Gamila's every move, reeling from the shock of the scolding that she'd just got.

Gamila was growing increasingly frustrated. Chris's knee was getting worse by the minute and this stupid woman was wasting precious time. Before Gamila could go in for the kill, a nurse who knew her walked by.

The nurse instantly knew something was wrong. She'd seen this perturbed expression on Gamila's face before, and it could only mean one thing—Gamila was letting someone have it . . . again.

"Hi Ms. Malone," said the nurse. "How is Chris doing tonight?"

"He has a knee bleed again. He needs to be treated immediately."

"Come on back. I'll have the nurse setup a room for you and Chris now. Do you have your medicine, or do we need to get some from the pharmacy?"

"I have the medicine. Tell them that they need to hurry because it's getting warmer and bigger. It's much worse than it was half an hour ago."

"I will make the doctor aware of his condition. Were you waiting long?" The nurse knew Gamila didn't usually tell them to hurry.

"It was twenty minutes before that woman behind the desk even acknowledged me. Chris's knee is bad and that woman doesn't seem to understand how serious this is. I told her Chris needed treatment immediately and it didn't register. She never even called the doctor. Anyway, this medicine seems to take time to work and they're always wasting my baby's time."

"I'm sorry about that," said the nurse.

"What are you sorry for? It wasn't you wasting our time."

"Well, I'm just sorry that you have to go through that routine process every time you come in."

"Routine? There was nothing routine about that process. She was rude, kept cutting me off, didn't listen, and doesn't seem to know how to do her job."

The nurse had heard all this before. She knew silence was her best option at that point.

The nurse's name was Kathy. She was one of the few nice nurses at The Hospital. Chris liked her, so she was all right in Gamila's book. Not to mention, Kathy was always all about business. She moved quickly when she had to, and she understood the seriousness of Chris's illness—especially a knee bleed.[3]

---

[3] One of the most frequent areas a bleed can occur in is the knee. The knee starts to feel tingly, hot, and tight. Once blood pools inside the knee or joint swelling occurs, the area gets tighter and hot to

* * *

Dwelling on a crisis or challenging ordeal was not Gamila's style, and she tried not to think too much about the negative aspects of their situation. Instead, she concentrated on getting the answers she needed regarding Chris's bleeding disorder—answers she wasn't getting from the doctors or nurses.

In the beginning, she didn't quite understand why her questions were never really answered. But as the number of treatments Chris needed increased, it became apparent that no one fully understands hemophilia.

Gamila began researching the rare disorder online and contacting relevant agencies and foundations. She also asked her sister to research all she could on hemophilia and bleeding disorders. As far as Gamila could tell, hemophilia seemed more complicated to the so-called experts than it did to her and her family.

Gamila and her sister got more information by doing their own research and talking to people than they did from The Hospital. They learned a lot. There was a time when hemophilia crippled anyone who suffered from it. Luckily, treatment options have

---

touch, and the pain is inescapable. If not treated immediately knee bleeds can cause serious or permanent damage. Source: www.hemophilia.org

advanced considerably since then. Today, people with bleeding disorders live full lives.

A common cause of death in individuals with a bleeding disorder used to be uncontrolled bleeding in the vital organs or bleeding from minor surgical procedures. In the 50s and 60s the life expectancy of hemophiliacs was only a measly twelve years. By the late 60s life expectancy had increased, but it was still less than twenty years.

Children with a bleeding disorder used to be given frozen plasma when they had a bleeding episode. The treatment was effective for minor bleeds, but the fresh plasma wasn't enough to control or subdue severe joint bleeds. As a result, many children with bleeding disorders suffered permanent damage to their knees and joints.

However, nothing compares to the tragedy of the late 70s to mid-80s. Over half of the people in the U.S. with hemophilia were infected with HIV[4] from contaminated donor blood from blood banks. It was finally determined in the 80s that HIV/AIDS can be transmitted through blood or plasma products, but

---

[4] HIV is a Human Immunodeficiency Virus infection where the virus attacks the cells in the immune system. There is no cure and as these cells replicate, they overwhelm the immune system and develop into full-blown acquired immunodeficiency syndrome (AIDS). Source: www.hemophilia.org/Bleeding-Disorders/Blood-Safety/HIV/AIDS

many individuals with hemophilia had already been infected.

* * *

By the time Chris was a year old he'd spent two hundred forty-nine days in The Hospital. And that didn't include the twenty-two days he'd spent in the hematology clinic for routine checkups.

The year had taken its toll on Gamila. Never mind that no one, including her, would've guessed that she'd be a mother at this stage of her life. The frustration had begun to show on her face, but she was a fighter. She'd had to familiarize herself with Chris's condition, understand the methods of his treatment, and fight off attackers who insisted on doing Chris more harm than good. And the fact that she did her own research, and came to her own conclusions, made her very unpopular at The Hospital.

Chris had just been in The Hospital a week ago, but they were back. Gamila looked up at the TV protruding from the wall attached to a thick black bracket. As she flicked through the channels her mind was consumed with thoughts of all the time Chris had spent there. A year isn't usually long enough to grow tired of a place—it can take that long just to get to know an environment—but Gamila had gotten to know this hospital a little too well.

She looked over at Chris. It was 1:20 a.m. and he was asleep. She thought about sneaking out of the room to get a snack from the vending machines on the first floor but she decided against it. She couldn't bear the thought of leaving Chris's side, not even for a moment.

The night nurse came into the room to check Chris's IV. "Is everything OK in here?"

"Yes," Gamila replied curtly.

The night nurse rolled her eyes and discreetly smacked her lips. By now, Gamila was an expert at tuning out their rudeness and sarcasm. Chris's fair skin, precious smile, and handsome features captivated the nurses' attention. They loved caring for him, but they despised Gamila and only spoke to her when it was absolutely necessary. But as long as they gave Chris his treatment, respected his space, and didn't get in her way, Gamila would ignore their crude, unprofessional behavior.

"Let me know if Chris needs anything," the nurse said as she smiled over the sleeping baby.

The night nurse practically collided with another nurse as she walked out of the room.

"Hey, you need to slow down," said the other nurse with a calm little laugh.

"Just trying to get away from that *B* in room 631." The night nurse pointed back at Chris's room.

"Who is it … Ms. Malone?" the other nurse whispered.

"You know it."

"Why is she so damn cold?"

"Something's probably stuck up her butt."

The nurses laughed as they headed for the nurses' station.

Gamila wasn't trying to listen, but she couldn't help hearing the part about "something's probably stuck up her butt." She didn't care. Whatever they said about her was of no concern. Gamila was only interested in getting the care and treatment her baby needed. Anyway, Gamila had already given that night nurse one tongue lashing, and she knew it was just a matter of time before she would have to give her another one.

* * *

Chris was on NovoSeven RT by the time he was almost two; it's given intravenously.[5] Around that same time, Chris's doctor told Gamila he wanted to discuss Chris's future treatment options with her.

---

[5]Intravenously means "through or within a vein." Source: www.dictionary.com/browse/intravenously

Gamila met with the doctor and he told her there was a possibility that Chris could "develop an inhibitor." Gamila had no idea what that meant and she began asking questions. Of course, trying to get information out of any of the doctors at The Hospital was like pulling teeth, but Gamila persisted until she was nearly satisfied with the doctor's vague response. He simply told her that if Chris developed an inhibitor it meant that his body was fighting off the treatment.

Then, the doctor got to the crux of the matter. He informed Gamila that Chris's only treatment option was to get a PICC line in his arm. The doctor said it would give them easier access when treating Chris, and it would allow for the continuous flow of medication to help fight the inhibitor.

Gamila didn't ever like hearing "only option." There are always other options, she thought. She wasn't going to make any decisions about Chris's future treatment until she had more information.

As always, Gamila wanted to make sure she understood all the implications of any new treatment or procedure before she consented. She wanted to know all the options, the common side effects, how it would affect Chris's life, and if it would affect his ability to make a living when he grew up. She felt that these were very reasonable questions that any concerned parent should ask. The doctors at The Hospital didn't share her sentiments.

Gamila did a little research and talked to other parents at the hematology clinic. She soon understood that "develop an inhibitor" meant that a body was recognizing the (coagulation recombinant) synthetic factor medication as a foreign substance and the antibodies in the immune system were trying to protect the body from the foreign substance. This made sense to Gamila. The medication is foreign, she thought.

She found out that the more factor you give a child at an early age, the higher the probability that the child will develop an inhibitor. She also learned that a PICC line—a peripherally inserted central catheter—is a long thin tube inserted through a vein in the patient's upper arm to administer medication for a long period of time.

Doctors wouldn't say how long Chris would need to keep the PICC line in his arm, but they indicated it could be years. That was lie number one.

Chapter Four

Angry & Frustrated

Gamila was labeled a "problem mother" at The Hospital because she dared to question them. She also made them explain the procedures and how medication would be administered to Chris. She didn't care what label they gave her, she only cared about the welfare of her child.

From talking to other parents in the hematology clinic, Gamila learned that no parent would recommend the PICC line or the Port-A-Cath.[6] Most parents told her that their child developed an infection and the PICC line eventually had to be removed. Some even felt their child's condition had gotten worse after the line was inserted.

---

[6] A port or Port-A-Cath is a small apparatus surgically implanted underneath the skin, usually in the upper chest area, and it connects to the vein. The port has a septum where the medication can be administered and blood can be drawn. Ports are commonly used in treating cancer patients.

Gamila was armed with this information the next time she saw one of Chris's doctors.

"Do you have any definitive information I can review about PICC lines?" she asked.

"You read too much," replied Dr. Way.

"That's not an *answer*."

"You need to just let us do our jobs. We are the professionals, not you." Dr. Way was visibly irritated.

"You guys keep saying that. And every time I ask for more information I get the runaround. I'm not just going to go along with whatever you say. I need to examine all available options and make sure I choose what's best for Chris."

"This is the only option. He needs to get a PICC line or a port. You don't seem to understand the importance of this for his care."

"No, *you* don't seem to understand the importance of his *health*. I'm trying to be patient with you doctors, but you're not making it easy for me. I've been following your suggestions, but *your* suggestions seem to keep my baby coming back to the hospital all the time."

"Well, it's obvious that you are not capable of making the decisions necessary to fully care for Chris."

"And what is that supposed to mean?" Gamila gave Dr. Way a penetrating stare.

Dr. Way began studying Chris's chart. She didn't know what else to say to this "problem mother."

The fact was that Dr. Way didn't want to answer Gamila because the doctor felt she didn't have to. As far as the doctors were concerned, Gamila needed to jump on their bandwagon or go somewhere else. Gamila wanted to go somewhere else plenty of times. The problem was that bleeding episodes are time sensitive and The Hospital was the closest hospital to her house. Gamila had no choice but to keep going there.

After a few minutes, Dr. Way finally said, "You should let us do our job. I am the professional. I am the one who went to medical school. I know how to deal with your child's condition, and I should know what is best for him."

"Yeah . . . you *deal* with it, but I *live* with it."

* * *

The doctors wouldn't take no for answer. They eventually started talking about "medical neglect" and Gamila knew she had no choice but to agree to try the PICC line. She was apprehensive, especially because Chris was only two years old. She was afraid he would pull it out by mistake or get curious and start messing with the tubing and cause a bleed.

Chris is right-handed and the doctors and Gamila agreed that the PICC line would be inserted in his left upper arm. That was lie number two.

Chris emerged from the surgical procedure with the PICC line not only in the wrong arm, but in the wrong place. It was in his right arm, in the crease between the upper arm and forearm where the arm bends. Because of this, they had to use masking tape to hold the tubing in place, similar to the way medical tape is used to hold an IV in place.

The doctor who performed the procedure was anxious when he went to talk to Gamila. "He's doing fine," the doctor kept repeating.

Gamila wasn't sure if the doctor was trying to convince himself or her. She knew the doctor wasn't telling her everything and she began probing him for more information. She finally learned that they had trouble waking little Chris. They had to give him medication to reverse the effects of the anesthesia.

Gamila's skeptical nature had proven invaluable. She had no doubt that they never would've told her the whole story if she hadn't persisted in her questioning. From the multiple misdiagnoses of her pregnancy to Chris's devastating circumcision to this procedure, Gamila had earned the right to be suspicious of them.

Chris wasn't really fazed by the PICC line. The idea was that it would make life simpler by making it easy to administer the medicine needed to reduce Chris's inhibitor. Gamila had her doubts, but she remained patient and hopeful.

It wasn't too long before the wrong placement of the PICC line started to become an issue. Being in the crease of Chris's right arm caused him to sweat around it much more than he would've if it had been put in his left upper arm as planned. And because Chris is right-handed, he used his right arm a lot, which caused him to sweat around the line even more. All this meant that the line had to be cleaned more frequently than usual.

The doctor advised Gamila to flush the line with heparin. She reminded the doctor that heparin thins the blood. Then she asked if it was a good idea to give heparin to a child with a bleeding disorder. The doctor told her she read too much and she should stop.

When your child is first diagnosed with a bleeding disorder doctors provide a few pamphlets for the parents to review. When the doctor told her to "stop," Gamila realized that she was supposed to read the material, but she wasn't supposed to comprehend anything or question them.

Chris eventually began complaining that the line was itching. And at times it got in his way and he would tug on it.

"No Chris, don't pull on it," Gamila would say.

"But it itches mommy, and it's in my way."

One day, after the line had been in for a couple of months, it was itching something fierce. Chris was scratching at it and blood suddenly sprayed out all over the place. Gamila looked at him. He was bewildered, staring at her with his innocent and enthusiastic brown eyes as if to say *Oops*. He'd scratched the tubing right out of his arm.

Gamila immediately rushed Chris to the hospital. She didn't even think about cleaning up the blood all over the floor and sofa.

After the wound was cleaned the doctors noticed that Chris was starting to get an infection at the insertion spot. Well that explains why it was itching so badly, Gamila thought.

Of course, the doctors claimed that an infection was unusual. They told her that the line could've stayed in Chris's arm for years if it had been inserted in the correct spot.

That was a pill Gamila didn't even bother trying to pretend to swallow. She'd already spoken with other parents and they all said the same thing—a few months after getting the PICC line, their child ended up with an infection.

* * *

Due to the risk of bleeds, hemophilia prevented Chris from playing like most kids. He spent the majority of his time sitting or in a hospital bed if he was recovering from a calf, knee, or joint bleed.

However, Chris wasn't a typical two-year-old in any way. His natural intelligence shined very early on and he made great use of his sitting time. He was reciting his ABCs before he was a year old. By age two he was learning to read. While he was learning to read, his aunt started teaching him math.

Even though Chris couldn't play sports, like most boys, he was—and still is—a sports fanatic. At two years of age he'd already mastered the art of playing video games. They let him play sports without risking a bleed and the games became his life.

Being Gamila's first child, and Gamila's mother's first grandbaby, people imagined that Chris would be spoiled beyond compare. Nothing could've been further from the truth. Gamila always made sure that he was clean, well dressed, and respectful. The nurses frequently commented on how neat he looked, and they were always pleasantly surprised at how well behaved a two-year-old could be. Chris's cool and calm demeanor was noticed by everyone—nurses, doctors, and other parents.

The doctors were so impressed with Chris that they asked Gamila for permission to use pictures of him in a few articles that were being written by a local medical school featuring the clinic's work and gene therapy research.

Chris was so advanced by the time he was two that he knew which medicine he needed and how much. He even knew which needle should be used to give it to him.

Unlike many babies and toddlers, Chris was never afraid of the needle. He didn't cry when his medicine was being administered and this fascinated the doctors and nurses. In fact, they couldn't believe it. They knew that someone was doing something wrong if Chris cried.

This was also extremely helpful to Gamila. She knew immediately which nurses would be allowed to treat her son simply by listening and watching his facial expressions. If he moaned, cried, or grimaced, the nurse had to go and no one could argue with her.

Gamila and Chris recalled one particular appointment at the hematology clinic. Chris was patiently sitting on the exam table, waiting to receive his treatment. He looked up as soon as the door squeaked open, and he remembers knowing immediately that something wasn't right.

The nurse walked into the examination room with a big smile and an even bigger syringe. She was excited to meet little Chris because she'd heard so much about him from the other nurses. She was told that he was very cooperative and a breeze to treat, especially for a two-year-old.

"OK, it's time for your medicine Chris," the nurse cheerfully announced.

Chris looked over at his mother. She was busy filling out yet another pile of paperwork and she wasn't watching the nurse. He looked at the nurse coming toward him and shouted, "Ooh, ooh, I think you made a *b-stake*." Chris tucked his hands under his legs and leaned away from the nurse.

Gamila glanced up. To her dismay, she noticed a huge 40cc syringe in the nurse's hand. "Have you lost your mind? You can leave now." Gamila didn't wait for a response before going back to her paperwork.

The nurse was confused. As she read Chris's chart it looked as though pure embarrassment was coursing through her veins like a lethal injection. She realized that she should've had a 23g or 25g butterfly needle[7]

---

[7] All the available products to treat hemophilia must be directly injected into the bloodstream. A butterfly needle, or winged infusion set, is one of the options to infuse the factor product into the

to administer factor VIII to a hemophilia patient, not a huge 40cc syringe. The nurse was clearly getting hot and she turned red. The woman was mortified and stuck to the spot she was standing on. She truly didn't know how to exit the room by that point.

Gamila looked up at the nurse once more. But this time, no words needed to be spoken. The nurse swallowed her embarrassment and walked out the door.

A few years later, Gamila was telling her sister about the incident. She said, "If Chris had been a grown man, he would've probably said, damn, you MFs are trying to kill me."

Eventually, only a handful of nurses were allowed to treat Chris. Fortunately, that was one thing that Gamila and the doctors agreed on.

---

bloodstream of people with hemophilia. Source: www.hemophiliafed.org/bleeding-disorders/hemophilia/treatment

Chapter Five

Family & Strangers

Most of Gamila's family learned early on to tread carefully when discussing Chris. Some family members thought she was being paranoid, but anything could be a potential threat to Chris's life. Many people didn't understand this, but his mother certainly did. Gamila had no choice but to be extremely cautious about absolutely everything pertaining to her son—from what he ate, to his activities, to what he wore, to his interaction with pets, to over the counter meds.

While researching all the meds that could not be given to a child with hemophilia, Gamila learned that anything containing aspirin was out of the question. In the 40s and 50s aspirin was given to hemophilia patients as a pain reliever, but aspirin is an NSAID—nonsteroidal anti-inflammatory drug—and a blood thinner. Patients with bleeding disorders cannot take aspirin or any NSAIDs. Basically, children with hemophilia can take Tylenol or acetaminophen for pain.

The list of off limits over the counter meds was lengthy, but Gamila took note of a few in particular.

Over-the-Counter Meds Containing Aspirin

Alka Seltzer	Midol Caplets
Fish Oils	Pepto-Bismol
Chewable Tabs	Pepto-Bismol Tablets
Heparin	Motrin
Duoprin-S Syrup	Excedrin

She wasn't surprised by the long list of medicine that Chris couldn't take. However, she was surprised by all the types of medication that contain aspirin, especially cough syrup.

A mouth bleed is one of the most severe bleeds for a child with hemophilia, and Gamila had to be very careful about the foods Chris ate. He couldn't have popcorn because the kernels could damage his gums and cause a bleed. Eating potato chips could lead to one of the chips poking his gums or getting stuck between his teeth, which could irritate his gums and cause them to swell or cause a mouth bleed. Hard candy can get stuck in anyone's teeth, but for someone with hemophilia this can result in a severe mouth bleed that can land that person in the hospital. And it wasn't just food that could cause Chris's mouth to bleed. Biting down on his lip or tongue by mistake would also cause a severe bleed.

Some people thought Gamila was being overprotective when they saw two-year-old Chris running around in a sturdy foam helmet. They never seemed to realize that these helmets are made specifically for head injury victims or children with disorders like hemophilia. The helmet had special padding inside to give added protection in the event Chris fell and hit his head. Toddlers fall down all the time and the helmet was a great investment. Chris also wore elbow pads and knee pads to protect him.

The helmet and pads, although necessary, were sometimes hard for Chris to bear. He would sweat underneath them, so he could only wear them for twenty to thirty minutes at a time. The sweat was a big problem, especially in cooler weather. Gamila didn't want sweat dripping from his head in case it might cause him to catch a cold or the flu.

When Gamila took Chris out in the helmet and pads she always got stares from neighbors, passersby, and other parents at the store or park. Most of the time she ignored their conspicuous looks. But on occasion, especially after another extended stay at The Hospital, she simply couldn't hold her tongue.

"Is there a problem?" Gamila asked a woman in the grocery store.

With a look of horror on her face, the woman stepped between her child and Gamila.

"Is there a problem?"

"No . . . no." The lady froze. She was obviously curious, and probably thinking that Gamila was an overprotective mom, but she couldn't take it when Gamila confronted her. "I was just . . ." She seemed to grow more nervous with every passing second.

"Then stop staring."

The mother turned and rushed toward her child. "Move it Zachary . . . go, keep walking."

"People are irritating. Just stop staring. Why do you act like you haven't seen a child in a helmet before? Children wear helmets and pads when they ride bikes, right?" Gamila was talking to herself. She didn't notice an elderly woman listening nearby.

"Yes, people are something else. If they want to know, they should just ask, not stare. It's impolite," said the elderly woman.

Gamila turned her head and looked down the aisle at the elderly woman. She looked pleasant. She was slightly hunched over and walking with a cane, but by no means fragile. Her eyes carried years of wisdom and experience. Gamila's demeanor changed and her anger started to subside.

"Yes, it is rude," said Gamila.

"He's a cutie." The elderly woman was focused on Chris.

"Thank you."

"And what's your name?" The lady bent over a little more and reached her hand out to Chris.

"Chris," he said, shaking her hand.

"Well, you said that nice and clear. Yeah, you understand what's going on very well." The woman smiled at him.

"People really shouldn't stare like that. He knows they're staring," said Gamila. "He gets these stares all the time. He has a condition where he has to wear this helmet for protection."

The elderly woman kept her eyes on Chris and continued smiling. "I'm sure he gets most of his stares because he's so handsome."

Gamila smiled. "Thank you."

"Your business is your business sweetie. Don't you let nobody come between that! Never mind what people think or say, it's how you perceive yourself is all that matters. That lady felt uncomfortable in your environment and she wanted you to feel uncomfortable too. You don't owe anyone an explanation, but I thank you for sharing. It will be better, you'll see." The elderly lady winked and smiled before she hobbled away.

Gamila smiled and watched the lady leave. Gamila's mind was calmed and she stood still for a bit. She knew the elderly lady was right. After her tranquil moment, Gamila grabbed Chris by the hand and finished her grocery shopping.

* * *

The steady growth of a child is usually a mother's dream. It means her child is healthy and developing as he or she should. But in Chris's case, his steady growth was both a great thing and a challenge. It was typical childhood growth that brought about most of his bleeds. The spontaneous joint bleeds were expected, but Chris's steady growth guaranteed him frequent visits to the hospital.

A lot of parents buy clothes for small children simply based on whether or not they fit, as anything else is immaterial. But Gamila wasn't so lucky. Certain clothes and shoes irritated Chris's skin and she had to learn fairly quickly which things he could and could not wear. This made clothes shopping for him quite tedious.

Once Chris started walking, the only shoes that didn't give him an ankle or foot bleed were Air

Jordan's. It would be an expensive shoe, Gamila thought. His feet grew like wildfire, and of course, the larger the shoe, the larger the price tag. Gamila often joked with her sister that she should send a letter to Jordan explaining her son's condition and asking for coupons or a free pair.

As Chris grew up, he had just about every pair of Jordan's Gamila could find. Some family members thought she was just being pretentious, or bougie. They had no idea that Gamila tried other shoes and all the other brands gave Chris an ankle bleed.

* * *

It was a cool day in November and Gamila, her cousin, and Chris were on their way to a doctor's appointment. Her car was suddenly struck on the driver's side, causing it to go into a tailspin. They would find out later that a taxi had run a red light.

Gamila and her cousin practically smashed into each other as their bodies were tossed around inside the vehicle. Once the cars came to a stop, Gamila's maternal instincts kicked in.

All she could think about was Chris. She instantly maneuvered herself into the back seat to get to him. Luckily, he was still safely secured in his car seat. She somehow managed to unstrap him and get out of the vehicle.

Gamila didn't know if her cousin was hurt, and she certainly didn't notice that her knee was bleeding. In fact, at first, she couldn't even tell anyone which car door she opened to get herself and Chris out of the wrecked vehicle. Her only concern was to examine Chris's body for injuries. He was a little shaken up, but he had no injuries that she could see.

Instead of going to the doctor, Gamila and Chris were once again headed back to the emergency room. But this time they arrived in an ambulance.

Chris had no visible injuries and no hot spots were forming in any of his joint areas, but the doctor treated Chris just to be on the safe side. Gamila was also treated.

After only four hours in the emergency room, both mom and baby were sent home.

Chapter Six

Politics

By 2001 Chris had worn a path to The Hospital. He was only four years old.

Despite the unsuccessful PICC line, doctors were still trying to persuade Gamila to let them fit Chris with a port. They maintained that the port would be better for Chris, and that not having it could be life-threatening. Those were lies three and four—and Gamila stopped counting.

She'd been given this same song and dance when they wanted Chris to get the PICC line. She'd expressed her concerns about the line at the time, and all her fears had come to pass. With the doctors now demanding that Chris undergo another procedure, Gamila was even more disinclined to comply. Not least because, unlike the PICC, where the tubing was inserted into Chris's arm, the port would have to be surgically implanted into his chest.

The doctors contended that a port would cut down on Chris's hospital visits. So Gamila started asking questions. How is the procedure done? How does the port connect to the vein? Chris has asthma, with the port being inserted into his chest, how will it affect his breathing? Her questions were never answered truthfully.

Gamila explained her grave concerns about the port but the doctors weren't interested. They blatantly told her that they believed she was just trying to be difficult. They informed her that she was the only parent at the clinic whose child hadn't tried the port. They also explained that the more patients they got to "participate," the more funding they would get, and more treatment options would become available in the future.

Gamila didn't care what the doctors thought about her. "I don't want to make life harder for my son. It's bad enough he has to be here every other day. I'm not going to add to his agony with something experimental."

Gamila was determined to act in the best interests of her child. If she wasn't convinced that the procedure would help Chris's condition, she wasn't going to consent.

*   *   *

Chris's knee had swollen up really badly. He and Gamila were back at the ER. His knee was so bad that it drew the attention of nurses, doctors, and other onlookers.

Gamila told the doctors she thought that the factor wasn't working any more, and she was right. They found out that Chris's body had become immune to NovoSeven and it was time for him to have another recombinant.

Chris was admitted to The Hospital and the doctors wasted no time before they started in on Gamila about implanting a port. Dr. Way gave Gamila vague and obscure information as always, but some of the others tried to broach the subject with a bit more flair, adding, "This is in the best interest of the child."

Gamila never left Chris alone in the hospital. She slept on the window seat in his room whenever he had to stay overnight. It had become her home away from home. If she needed to go home she made sure her sister or Chris's dad could stay with him until she returned. Gamila's sister sometimes insisted that she needed to take a break and go home for a bit, but Gamila didn't like to do that—even when her sister was right. Gamila knew the doctors and nurses like the back of her hand, and she also knew that she was the best qualified person to deal with them.

Gamila was resting her head on the back of the padded window seat when Dr. York came in and sat down beside her. Dr. York was trying to make the port sound more appealing. Her more, subtle manipulation may have worked—on a new mother of a different caliber.

"We know you only want the best care for your son, and we know you're exhausted from the frequent hospital stays," said Dr. York in a relaxed monotone.

Gamila didn't have the inclination or the energy to fight that day. Dr. York was one of the nicer doctors and Gamila felt comfortable explaining her concerns to the doctor, again. She felt Dr. York at least listened to her, even if her concerns weren't really taken into consideration.

Dr. York listened attentively before further elaborating the ostensible benefits of the port. She said she understood Gamila's concerns and repeated that she knew Gamila was worn out from the frequent hospital stays. Then she added, "The port will alleviate most of that." Dr. York stood up. "Just think about it Ms. Malone. It will help you and Chris in the long run. It's a simple procedure and it doesn't take long."

"I'll think about it," Gamila said. She laid the back of her neck against the top of the cushion, careful not to hit her head on the faux marble windowsill as she had done before.

Dr. York felt that she'd finally made some headway with Ms. Malone. Little did she realize that Gamila had already thought about it. She'd been thinking about the port since it was first mentioned to her when Chris was two years old. She'd made up her mind then and the answer was still no.

The doctors hadn't convinced Gamila that Chris did in fact suddenly need a port. But they had let it slip that the clinic stood to benefit financially if she allowed them to do the procedure on her son. Putting Chris through an unnecessary surgical procedure was not Gamila's idea of care. The other thing was that Dr. Way had told her that the surgeon would implant the device through Chris's arm, but Gamila found out that a Port-A-Cath is implanted via a vein in the neck. Any surgical procedure is risky for a child with hemophilia, and Gamila had to be damn sure her child truly needed it before she would consent.

Gamila could barely keep her eyes open the next morning. Sleep was hard to come by in The Hospital. Not only did she have to keep an eye on the nurses and doctors, she also had to run Chris back and forth to the restroom. This was normal any time he was unable to walk, but carrying a four-year-old pushing over forty pounds wasn't an easy task. Not to mention, he was nearly as tall as Gamila.

"You gonna be bigger than mommy in a minute Chris," said Gamila as she hauled him onto her back for another trip to the toilet.

Chris smiled with glee and said, "Yep."

They both laughed. Gamila put him on the toilet and leaned against the restroom wall. She looked at his knee. It was finally getting better. "We should be able to go home in a day or two buddy."

"Yes!" Chris excitedly waved his hands in the air and a huge grin overtook his face.

Chris tried to stand up when he was done. Gamila caught him and put him back on the seat.

"No man, not yet," said Gamila. "You're not ready to walk yet. OK?"

"OK."

He waited patiently for Gamila to rest for a few seconds more before she helped him off the toilet and carried him back to his bed.

"Is it OK if mommy goes downstairs for a minute to get something from the cafeteria?"

"Sure," he said. His words were short and sweet, just like his mother's.

Gamila was leery about leaving Chris, even for a moment. She wanted to wait to go to the cafeteria until he went back to sleep, but that was a coin toss. One of the side effects of the factor medication is that it may keep a patient up all night, and the next day too.

Gamila finally hit the call button. The nurse stopped in her tracks when she saw Gamila.

"Oh, I'm sorry. Did you call for a nurse?" The nurse acted as if she was in the wrong room. She backed out into the hallway and checked the room number.

Gamila wanted to laugh at the nurse's hesitation, but she was too exhausted. "Yes, it was me."

"Oh, OK." The nurse gave a nervous little laugh. "How can I help?"

"I'm running down to the cafeteria on the first floor and I need you to keep an eye on Chris," said Gamila.

"All right."

"He should be fine for now, but he may have to go to the restroom. In that case, you'll need to carry or wheel him in there."

"I understand," said the nurse.

"Under no circumstances can you leave him alone in the restroom. If there's an accident or something, he can't reach that call button in there," Gamila said.

"OK, I got it. I will take good care of Chris," the nurse said enthusiastically.

Gamila went downstairs and returned as quickly as possible. When she stepped out of the elevator the nurses' station and hallway were oddly silent. Too silent, thought Gamila.

She hurried down the hall to Chris's room. Gamila heard Chris's distinctive cry before she reached the door. "Oh my goodness, what's happened?" Her heart descended into the pit of her stomach and her blood started to boil. She ran in the room and before she could say anything the silly nurse started to speak.

"I just left him in the restroom for a second. Just a quick second. I told him not to get up but he got up anyway."

"I told you to stay in the restroom with him. I told your ass that. You people don't ever listen. This is ridiculous. Go get the head nurse and the doctor on duty. Simple. Just simple." Gamila was furious.

"I only left for a second," the nurse said again.

"I don't care to hear your explanation. He's a child who's been in bed for a month. You think he wasn't going to try and walk? That's what your sorry butt was there for, to make sure he stayed off his feet." Gamila looked at Chris's knee. It was getting bigger again. She touched it and it was warming up fast. "Just stop talking and looking stupid and go get the damn doctor."

The other nurses just stood around gawking. They didn't want to get in the middle of this, but they never wanted to miss the wrath of Ms. Malone. Some couldn't believe the nurse left an injured four-year-old alone in a restroom, let alone one with a bleeding disorder. The instructions Gamila left for her were explicit, but the nurse had her own ideas. Even so, leaving a handicapped child alone certainly wasn't protocol.

The doctor examined Chris. It was determined that he had an acute fracture in his knee from the fall. This unexpected setback left Chris and Gamila in The Hospital for an additional two months.

Rather than holding the nurse accountable for her actions, the doctors swarmed Chris's hospital room trying to convince Gamila that if Chris had the port the accident could've been prevented. They were turning the tables to cover-up their mistake. Gamila expected nothing less, but this was altogether different. This time, her son had been injured.

Gamila knew she had to seek another opinion about the port, and fast. She never imagined that The Hospital was about to make her fight to keep her children.

Chapter Seven

In the Best Interests of My Child

The Hospital insisted that Chris was now facing a life or death situation. They said catastrophe was just around the corner if he didn't get the port.

The only catastrophe Gamila could see would be letting The Hospital inflict another ill-fated treatment on her son. She was determined to get a second opinion about the port.

It usually took months to be seen at another medical center, but Gamila managed to get an appointment for Chris the following month. The center was about twenty minutes farther from her house than The Hospital, but the extra distance didn't matter. She had to get a second opinion. Meanwhile, she would continue taking Chris to the hematology clinic at The Hospital for his treatments.

The next time Gamila shuffled through the doors of the clinic with Chris, the nurse told her that he couldn't be seen that day. Gamila was confounded.

She informed the nurse that Chris had another bleed and reminded her how important it was for him to be treated right away, but to no avail.

Gamila was demanding to know why they were refusing to treat Chris when Dr. Way appeared from behind a door. The doctor made it clear to Gamila that if she didn't cooperate with their treatment plans, then Chris could no longer be seen at their facility.

"What am I supposed to do?" Gamila was incredulous. "He has a bleed. I thought it was imperative that his bleeds are treated immediately."

"You are the only parent who refuses to get the port and you are being difficult, so we can't see you here," Dr. Way said. "You'll need to go to the ER."

Gamila couldn't believe they were refusing to treat her baby, but Chris needed his medication and she didn't have time to argue with the doctor. Gamila grabbed her bags, picked Chris up off the chair, and left.

It was frustrating enough that Gamila and Chris had to make regular trips to the ER when the hematology clinic was closed, but to go just for a regular treatment was ridiculous. She made her way down to the ER, rolling her eyes in anticipation of the usual madness.

Precious time had already been wasted and Chris's bleed was getting warmer. It's a good thing I always carry extra ice packs, Gamila thought. She knew the wait time in the ER would be ridiculous and the whole thing would be overwhelmingly frustrating. She gritted her teeth, took a deep breath, and mentally prepared herself to deal with their dysfunction.

As they waited to be seen, Gamila remembered another time she took Chris to the ER and the receptionist suddenly decided she wanted to be more than a receptionist. Gamila had waited as long as she could, but a bleed had to be treated as quickly as possible, and they were running out of time.

Gamila got up and stood in front of the reception desk. The receptionist was talking with another mother. Gamila overheard the conversation and realized that the other mother's child was in for a cold.

"I'm sorry to interrupt," said Gamila, "but my son really needs to see a doctor. I'm not saying that your daughter's health is less important, but my son is bleeding internally."

The other mother looked at Gamila with grave concern. "No, please, go ahead."

"You can't just cut in front of people!" shouted the receptionist.

"No, it's OK. I don't mind," said the caring mother. "He's bleeding internally. Please, let her go ahead of me."

"How can I help you?" the receptionist asked with a sneer.

"My son has hemophilia, a bleeding disorder," said Gamila. "He needs to be treated right away."

"He has pretty nasty bruises on his leg," said the receptionist. "Where did they come from?"

"I don't know. He has spontaneous bleeding all the time. Look, he needs to see a doctor right away."

"So you *don't know* how he got those bruises?" The receptionist's tone was getting worse. "Did he fall out of a tree, or fall down or something? How can you *not know* where those bruises came from?"

"Look, just let us go to the back so my son can get treated," said Gamila. She was tired and didn't have the energy to answer the receptionist's questions or accusations.

The receptionist made a call. As soon as she hung up she said, "The nurse will be out to get you."

Gamila moved to the side of the reception desk to wait for the nurse. The sliding doors opened as Gamila was examining Chris's knee. She glanced up and saw the social worker. The social worker went to the reception desk and briefly spoke with the receptionist.

"That's her over there." The receptionist pointed at Gamila. "Her son has bruises all over him and she *doesn't know how they got there.*"

The social worker looked at Gamila and Chris and smiled. "Well hello Chris. You guys back again, huh?" She turned to the receptionist. "Yes, Chris has hemophilia which is a bleeding disorder. Mom may not know where the bruises came from. Children with hemophilia have spontaneous bleeding episodes." The social worker waved her hand, signaling Gamila to follow her. "Come on to the back and let's get you taken care of."

The receptionist's jaw dropped. She thought she was reporting a case of child abuse and her accusation bit her on the ass.

Misconceptions like this happen all the time to parents of children with hemophilia. The receptionist jumped to conclusions and wasted valuable time. She prolonged Chris's bleeding because she didn't listen and she'd decided to be more than a receptionist that day.

These unsettling memories played over and over in Gamila's head as she endured the long wait in the ER. They'd been coming here for years, but most of the staff were still clueless about bleeding disorders.

Going through the ER was a time crusher, and any delay in getting treatment meant more pain and suffering for Chris. The time it took to get Chris's treatment that day put him back in The Hospital.

The stay was like every other time. Gamila slept on the window seat in the room on the fifth floor and watched over Chris as he healed. By the fourth day, Gamila needed to go home to change clothes and take a breather.

As she approached the front door of her house she noticed a business card stuck between the screen door and the doorframe. She read the card: Child Protective Services Division.

Gamila paused before pushing through her front door. She laid the card on the dining room table. As she headed upstairs to shower her mind began racing, trying to figure out why CPS would be at her door.

When she got out of the shower she noticed the blinking red light on the answering machine in her bedroom. She pressed the button and, lo and behold, there were a number of messages from the child services lady. The last one was:

> We've left you five messages now. We are beginning to think you are avoiding this situation. You will leave me no choice but to remove the children from the home if I cannot get a response from you.

Gamila was livid. She knew The Hospital must've reported her, but she couldn't understand their justification for doing such a thing. Since the clinic had turned her away and refused to treat Chris, she'd assumed that she wouldn't have to be bothered with them again.

Slick asses, thought Gamila. They kicked us out on purpose. . . to give themselves a reason to call CPS. Gamila knew she couldn't waste any more time at the house. She had to get back to Chris.

As soon as Gamila got back to The Hospital she was inclined to head straight for the hematology clinic, but she decided against it. She needed to talk to the CPS lady.

Gamila phoned the social worker from CPS. She wanted to know who called CPS and why. She carefully listened to what the CPS lady had to say. The social worker indicated that the hematology clinic submitted a complaint of medical neglect. The complaint detailed a number of specifics:

- Child needs to get a port due to a life-threatening situation.
- Mom has had transportation issues.
- No call, no show for appointments.
- Refuses to follow medical advice and ignores

treatment plans.

- Mom isn't responsible enough to make the proper decisions for her son's care.
- Frequent ER visits.

Gamila couldn't believe what she was hearing. She was stunned by the allegations, but she was far from surprised at who initiated the complaint.

In her defense, Gamila replied to the CPS lady with a number of points:

- First of all, if you were doing *your* job, you would have realized that we've been in the hospital for the past four days.
- Secondly, there is no medical neglect. I refuse to allow The Hospital to use my son as a guinea pig for their experimental treatment. I know the port has been put in many people, some children, but they have not proven that it is *medically necessary* for *my* son. I simply asked them for more information and if I could get a second opinion.
- My son has a severe bleeding disorder and any surgical procedure would be detrimental to his health. They know that, but they don't care.
- No call, no show? Please. Are they serious? The

only time I wasn't able to make it to a doctor's appointment was when we were in a car accident, and instead of going to the doctor's appointment we had to go to the ER. Makes sense, right?

- We did miss another appointment after we were released from the emergency room at 5 a.m. The doctor's appointment was scheduled for 8 a.m. and we wouldn't have made that one because we were exhausted from being in the ER all night. Furthermore, the doctors typically come down to the ER and see Chris when he's there. I wouldn't have thought he needed to be seen again three hours later.

- Speaking of ER visits, the clinic turned us away and refused to treat my son. They said we weren't allowed in their clinic anymore and I had to take Chris to the ER from now on. So why are they concerned with my son's well-being now?

- I have never had transportation problems that aren't common.

- Now, before you go threatening people, perhaps you may want to check out the facts.

The CPS lady was apologetic by that point. She agreed to make a trip to The Hospital to discuss the matter further with Gamila.

Before the CPS lady spoke to Gamila, she spoke to numerous witnesses at The Hospital, including some nurses. Everyone confirmed most of what Gamila had said. The CPS lady also retrieved Chris's hospital and hematology clinic records. According to the hematology clinic's records:

- The patient (Chris) is always clean and neat in appearance.
- Mom is attentive, eager to learn, and Chris is the same.
- Chris's aunt brought him in today. He is well-dressed and his aunt is neat in appearance as well.
- Child seems happy and energetic.
- Mom refuses to get the port, life-threatening!

The CPS lady noticed that the last note was made the day before the complaint was lodged. She realized the clinic had fabricated a little of the story.

Gamila wasn't out of the woods yet. Once a CPS case is opened, it remains open for six months, even if the allegations are unfounded. The Hospital knew exactly what they were doing, Gamila thought. *They're trying to bully me into getting the port, and they're willing to use ruthless tactics.*

The doctors thought they were putting Gamila in an impossible position, but she was a fighter. She was not going to allow them to take her children, or to dictate Chris's treatment.

* * *

As the date for the appointment at the other medical center neared, Gamila was filled with high hopes. Those were dashed as soon as she walked in and saw one of the ER doctors from The Hospital. When the doctor saw Gamila, her heart sank too.

The doctor was well aware of the reason for Gamila's visit to the medical center. Gamila didn't even bother asking her how she knew.

They gonna take my kids, Gamila thought. She felt beaten, but not defeated. She knew she had to keep fighting for Chris's sake.

"To be honest," said the doctor, "Chris is one of the best hemophilia patients I've seen. He has use of all his limbs and his mobility's good. Aside from the knee issues, he's doing pretty well."

"Yeah, his knee keeps getting reinjured, even when he's in The Hospital," Gamila stated matter-of-factly.

The doctor was vague and rather distant after that. It was obvious that she didn't want to get involved in this mess. She didn't want her name associated with any lawsuits and she wanted to keep the meeting as clean as possible.

The doctor didn't realize that Gamila just wanted a second opinion. She wasn't out to try and sue The Hospital for their mistakes or medical neglect, she just wanted to obtain the best care for her child.

"Well," said the doctor, "It doesn't seem life-threatening and I'm not going to say Chris needs the port. However, I'm not going to say he doesn't need it."

Gamila gave the doctor a stern look. "Thank you for your time." She stood up, grabbed Chris, and walked out of the examination room. Wow, this was a waste of time. You are all in this together, thought Gamila.

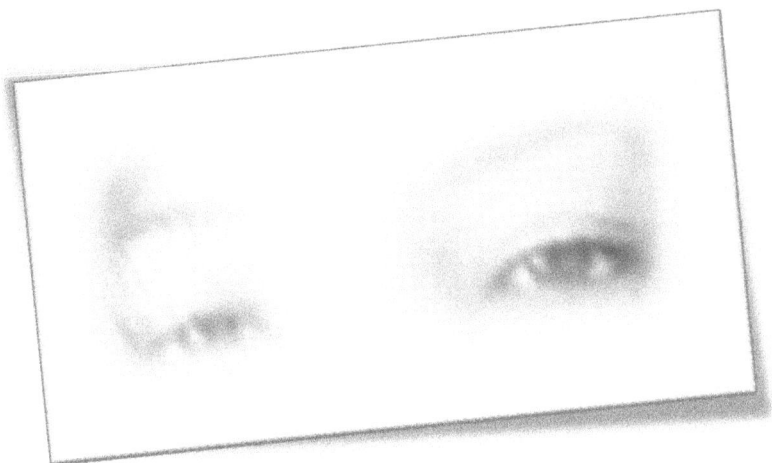

LIFE'S OPTIONS

Chapter Eight

Finally, A Better Way

Chris's fifth birthday was approaching fast and everything was weighing heavily on Gamila. Not only did she need better information and better medical advice, Chris would be starting school soon and she needed the help and guidance of a physician who truly cared about his well-being.

Gamila was able to get an appointment for Chris at one of the best treatment care centers in Michigan—a big hospital with an even bigger reputation. It was ranked number one in the state and in the nation. The University Hospital was about an hour away from their house, but Gamila was desperate. She would do anything to protect her children, and the first thing she needed to do was resolve this "life or death" situation. If she had to drive an hour to do it, she would find a way to make it work.

As they sat in the examination room waiting for the doctor, she prepared herself for another uphill battle. Gamila was going over her concerns in her head, and she was trying to figure out how she could make this new doctor understand that she was simply seeking options for Chris. She was trying to remain optimistic, hoping this visit would be better than her visit to the medical center.

Dr. Mint entered the room with a pleasant smile. Sincere caring and dedication were written all over his face. Gamila immediately felt his warmth. She knew her worries were over.

"Well hey there little guy. You look good. Life or death situation, really?" Dr. Mint asked Chris to have a seat on the bed. The doctor probed him for a bit, examining his limbs and joints. "I gotta say, he's one of the best hemophilia patients I've seen in a while. Aside from his knee issues, all of his joints seem to be in pretty good shape. So what's the problem?"

"The Hospital said that he has to get the port and that there are no other options," said Gamila.

"Well, there are always options. They may be limited, but you certainly have options."

"I just don't want Chris to endure more pain and trouble than he already has."

"That's certainly understandable." Dr. Mint stared at Chris for a moment. "Have they talked to you about treating him at home?"

"They first talked to me about treating Chris at home when he was a year old. But I was a new mom and I wasn't ready then. Plus, they knew very little about hemophilia so, obviously, I was reluctant. Anyway, I've taken the classes and completed all the necessary paperwork now, but The Hospital insists he needs the port and they said I can't treat him at home."

"Well, I don't think he needs the port, for one. Secondly, are you looking for a second opinion or a new doctor altogether?"

"Both." Gamila was there for a second opinion, but she had it in her mind that she would find another hematology clinic. "I want to get out from underneath The Hospital and I would love to find a new hematology clinic. My son's condition seems to be getting worse under their care, and they're causing us more trouble than we need."

"OK, I can take Chris as a new patient. Do you want to start treating him at home?"

"Yes." Gamila was getting a little excited. She'd learned to be prepared for the rug to be pulled out from under her, and she'd been half-expecting CPS or a social worker to walk through the door at any moment. She was surprised that this visit was going so well.

Dr. Mint smiled at Gamila. "OK, let me call in one of the nurses and test your skills." He opened the exam room door and called for one of the nurses. He left the door ajar and turned to Gamila. "Now, have you tested out your skills at home, or in another facility?"

"Well, I poked on my cousin a few times. Each time I got a blood return. Of course my cousin was so silly, when he saw the blood travel through the tubing he would pretend to pass out."

The doctor and Gamila were sharing a laugh as the nurse walked in.

"Sounds like you guys are having fun. Well look at him, he is so handsome." The nurse smiled as her eyes focused on Chris. He smiled back. She turned to the doctor and whispered, "He looks good. He has hemophilia?"

"Yes, I was telling his mom that he is a pretty good-looking patient. His joints are good and his limbs are good. He's got minor bruising but nothing major."

Using the nurse as a patient, Dr. Mint had Gamila walk him through a treatment. Gamila's test was successful and he said she was ready. He gave her all the necessary paperwork and information she needed to treat Chris at home.

Gamila couldn't believe it. She didn't even have to say any of the things she'd rehearsed in her mind. Dr. Mint simply examined Chris, made his determination, and stood by his own findings.

Chapter Nine

The Home Care Factor

When Gamila began treating Chris, a home care nurse would visit to make sure everything was going well, and sometimes the nurse showed her different or new techniques. Gamila learned so much while Chris was under the care of Dr. Mint, and he was pleased with the excellent care she was giving Chris at home. Gamila eventually received phlebotomy, or venipuncture training, and she became certified in CPR with AED Heartsaver® First Aid.

One winter, in the midst of a blizzard, Chris was running low on his factor VIII medication. The home care agency had missed filling his prescription, but it wasn't a problem because Gamila had enough medicine to last until the weather improved.

The agency was concerned to make sure Chris got his prescription. They apologized profusely to Gamila and told her that they were dispatching a courier to deliver the medication to her doorstep. The snow was nearly two feet high by then, and there were special alerts to keep off the roads. Gamila told them the weather was too bad and said it wasn't necessary for them to make the delivery that day, but the agency insisted.

It took the courier over an hour and a half to reach Gamila's place. The snow in the huge apartment complex's parking lot was deep, and it wasn't long before the courier's car was stuck. When he got out of the car he saw that one of his front tires had been swallowed by a mound of snow.

Not wanting to delay the delivery any longer, the courier pulled the big box from his back seat and continued on foot. He trudged through the snow for what seemed like three miles before he finally reached Gamila's building. His hands felt frozen inside his thick gloves as he rang the doorbell.

Gamila quickly ran downstairs to open the door. She was shocked at the sight of the courier. Snowflakes covered the shoulders of his coat and the top of his hat, his eyes were running, his nose was red, and his cheeks were flushed.

The courier stepped inside and took a deep breath. "Sorry I'm late." His teeth were chattering. "My car got stuck in the entrance way so I had to walk around to your building."

"Oh my goodness. Are you OK? Do you want some coffee, something hot to drink? Please, come upstairs and warm up before you go out in this mess again."

"Oh, thank you ma'am, but I must be going." He smiled, handed her the paperwork for her signature, and regained his composure before heading back out the door.

When he stepped outside he realized his car was much closer than he thought. The apartment complex was pretty much arranged in a circle. Gamila's building—building number twenty—was only two buildings away from the front entrance. On his walk in, the courier started at building one and walked all the way around. "Dang, I could've gone this way before. Oh well, here we go!"

He started pushing through the high snow, moving as rapidly as he could. He hadn't even thought about how he was going to get his car out. He heard footsteps crunching in the snow behind him.

"Hey, courier guy, wait! Gamila sent me to help you! Wait!" a deep voice shouted. The guy's nose was running and he was slightly out of breath when he caught up to the courier. He waited a moment to catch his breath. "Hey man, Gamila sent me to help you get your car out of the snow. I'm her cousin, Lyonell. I didn't know what you needed so I brought these." Lyonell held up a shovel and rock salt. "Maybe we can create some friction under the tires and get you unstuck."

"Good idea." The courier was relieved. "Thanks, I appreciate it."

Chapter Ten

School & Chris

The transition from hospital treatments to home treatments was smooth. With the support of Dr. Mint, and having found the right home care agency, Gamila finally felt a sense of relief. Now, rather than battling over Chris's care, she could concentrate on raising him.

The next hurdle for Chris was school. A bump on the head or a fall during recess could be life-threatening. In fact, many normal things and routine procedures could cause extra trouble for Chris. When he was five he had a tooth pulled and his gums didn't respond well to the pressure. The dentist couldn't stop the bleeding and Chris eventually had to have a blood transfusion.

The other thing Gamila had to consider was that Chris was growing fast. This caused frequent spontaneous bleeding episodes—mostly joint bleeds—and on occasion the bleeds could temporarily put him in a wheelchair. Gamila knew Chris would have to miss a lot of school because of the spontaneous bleeds, and by law, the school would have to report his absences. She seriously considered homeschooling, but she tossed out that idea because she didn't want Chris to feel any more alienated or isolated than he may have already felt because of his condition.

Gamila researched her options. She discovered that she could protect Chris's right to an education under Section 504 of the *Rehabilitation Act of 1973* and the *Individuals with Disabilities Education Act (IDEA)*.[8] She applied to the state to have Chris recognized as child with a disability. This would allow him to miss as many days of school as necessary due to his illness.

Before Chris started school, Gamila consulted with his doctor. The doctor agreed that the school needed to be aware of Chris's condition. The University Hospital sent a nurse and a representative to meet with the principal, school nurse, and teachers.

The nurse from the hospital explained to the school staff that it was imperative for them to act quickly if Chris was injured. She told them it was necessary to examine the injured area, test to see if it

---

[8] Source: www2.ed.gov/about/offices/list/ocr/docs/edlite-FAPE504.html

was hot, and immediately apply ice. Then she showed them a video that explained bleeding disorders in further detail. After the video, some of the teachers were discreetly crying in sympathy. However, other teachers asked whose classes Chris would be in, and if he wasn't going to be in one of their classes they were counting their lucky stars.

Gamila was of course nervous sending Chris off to school, but he enjoyed it. From a very early age it was obvious that he's exceptional. By the time Chris started kindergarten, he was already writing his name, reading at a first grade level, and studying multiplication. Once the teachers realized that Chris wasn't a problem child, and that he was a great student, they were happy to have him in their classes.

His first year of school went well, aside from a time when he was accidently shoved into a locker in the hallway. The handle on the locker gave him a bleed in the center of his back. Chris missed three days of school, but it took over a week for him to heal. Gamila was allowed to pick up his assignments and drop them back off so he didn't fall behind on his schoolwork.

Chris's school eventually began using the Internet and an online gateway for K-12 students and parents. It was a great way of sharing school information, and it also allowed the teachers to upload Chris's assignments. Whenever he was out due to his illness, he could just print the assignments and submit his completed work through the school's student portal.

Most of the time Chris didn't even bring homework home because he'd finish it in class. Gamila could probably count on one hand the number of times Chris actually brought books home from school for the purpose of doing homework or studying. It wasn't until years later, when he was in his senior year of high school and struggling with Calculus II that he had to hit the books outside school.

After several years, the school nurse and Chris's teachers became more familiar with his condition. His intelligence and dedication put him in the spotlight, and the teachers were fond of him. Teachers began asking, "Chris, you taking my class next year?" Chris, always the calm and consummate gentlemen, would simply smile and agree.

The biggest challenge for Chris wasn't learning, it was concealing his condition. He missed anywhere from sixty to ninety days of school a year due to bleeding episodes. Chris didn't want anyone to know why because he didn't want to be treated differently. After he'd missed days, or even weeks, he'd just tell his classmates he'd been sick.

Since Chris couldn't play sports or participate in physical education classes, Gamila discussed alternatives with his teachers. He played in the elementary school band, and from first through fourth grades he was a member of the student council.

When Chris came home one day and told his mom he needed a résumé she thought he was joking. He was ten years old. He explained that he was trying to get a job at school and she figured it was just a school project. Once she read the documentation she realized it was true. The school wanted to promote responsibility and real world accountability. There was a real bank—Citizens' Bank—in Lighthouse Elementary School, and students could open accounts and deposit and withdraw money. The school made several banking positions available to students, but they had to apply and interview for the jobs.

Chris's auntie helped him with a résumé, and the day of his interview he wore a tie and dress slacks to school. After several weeks of interviewing kids for the positions, the principal would announce who got the jobs.

The day finally came when the principal arrived in Chris's classroom. The class was silent. The kids' eyes widened as they eagerly awaited the principal's announcement.

"This was supposed to be a fun and rewarding experience, but I thought you guys would take it seriously. I guess I was wrong," said the principal. "You'll be moving on to middle school soon, and these are the kinds of things you'll eventually have to learn. With that said, there was one student who truly impressed me and my staff. He was well dressed and well-prepared for his interview. He took the interview seriously, and for that I am giving him the position of branch manager."

"Hey, I didn't know we were going to be working, like, for real," one kid shouted from the back of the classroom.

"OK Brian, that's rude," said the teacher. "And yes, the positions are very real. The idea is that kids will be working in the bank here on campus."

"The new branch manager of the Citizens' Bank is Chris Malone," the principal said as he smiled and walked over to shake Chris's hand.

Chris smiled. He was excited about his new position. He couldn't wait to go home and tell his mom. The job kept him busy. He worked in the morning, during physical education class, and in the afternoon before school ended.

That was just the beginning for Chris. All his teachers admired him, and they were amazed that he never used his condition as an excuse for not completing his assignments or not applying himself to his extracurricular activities.

From the time he was a toddler, Chris has loved sports—football, basketball, golf, tennis, he watched them all. Once he reached his adolescent and teenage years, he concentrated more on basketball and football. He knew he would never be able to play football, but he thought perhaps, one day, he would be able to play basketball. He tried playing a few times, because he wanted to feel some sense of normalcy, but playing gave him knee bleeds.

By the time Chris went to high school he didn't have to worry so much about concealing his condition from his fellow students. If he'd been absent, or was limping, most of them would just say, "That darn basketball injury, ahh man!" And Chris would simply agree and keep walking.

Chapter Eleven

Spontaneous Episodes

Whether Chris was going across town or out of town, his condition meant that he and his mom always had to be prepared for eventualities. And they always had to take extra things with them.

Gamila never left the house without plenty of ice packs, alcohol wipes, surgical gloves, and Chris's medications—a nebulizer for his asthma and his factor VIII replacement therapy (recombinant). It was difficult to keep Chris's medical alert bracelet current because he was on several different recombinant medications over the years, so Gamila carried a letter from the doctor explaining his condition. She also made sure to have snacks and a change of clothes with her. If Chris left the house in jeans and got a knee bleed he would have to change into shorts, and if he got an elbow or arm bleed he'd have to put on a short-sleeved shirt. This was to prevent his clothes from irritating the bleed area.

* * *

The kids were excitedly preparing for another summer road trip with their auntie. They were heading down to Austin, Texas to spend a few weeks with their grandmother. Gamila's sister usually drove from Dallas, Texas to Michigan to pick up the kids and drive them back to Texas. Once Gamila's sister told her she was on her way, Gamila had about twenty-two hours to get everyone and everything together.

Gamila had to make sure she had a current letter from the doctor explaining Chris's condition, and she had to have a power of attorney prepared so her sister could make medical decisions for Chris while he was in her care. Gamila also had to make arrangements with the home care agency to ship the next month's medication to Texas, and for a home care nurse to give him his treatments there. And then, of course, she had to pack the usual stuff for the kids, and all the extras for Chris—ice packs, extra clothes, and plenty of medication.

Chris and his little sister A'zha had only been at their grandmother's house a week when Chris got a knee bleed. Grandma had Chris put ice on his knee, and then she just waited for the home care nurse to arrive. The nurse never showed up and Chris's grandma seemed to think his knee would miraculously get better on its own.

A'zha was six at the time. She was getting frantic. "I think you should call my momma."

"Is the ice working?" asked their grandmother.

"No," said Chris. His knee was getting bigger and hotter and the pain was getting worse. The longer the bleed, the more pain the patient suffers. Chris knew he had to do something.

Chris called his mother in Michigan. She immediately knew from the sound of his voice that something was terribly wrong. He explained that his knee was swollen, hot, and painful.

"The home care nurse didn't make it out there to you today?" Gamila was trying to hide her frustration.

"No."

"OK. Let me try and call her again."

Gamila stared at her computer as she listened to the ringing on the other end of the phone. The call went to voicemail. Gamila was furious. She called the home care service but she got their voicemail too. She leaned back in her chair and looked over at the clock on the kitchen wall. It was 2 p.m. and she couldn't understand why no one was answering the phone at the home care service.

Gamila knew Chris had no time to wait for the home care nurse, and she could visualize what a disaster it would be if she had her mother take Chris to the hospital. Hemophilia is rare, and you really need to know how to get around the red tape and lengthy hospital questionnaire to move on to the treatment phase. Gamila figured that their wait time in an ER would be just as long as it would take her to fly to Austin.

She called Chris back as she simultaneously looked online for the next flight to Texas. She scrolled down the list of flights from Detroit Metropolitan Airport to Austin-Bergstrom International Airport. There was a flight leaving at 4:05 p.m., arriving in Austin at 7:25 p.m. Central time.

Gamila lived about forty-five minutes from the airport and she had to move fast. She grabbed a small carry-on bag and filled it with essentials, telling Al, "We need to go!"

He didn't ask questions. He simply got up and helped her through the door. It wasn't until they were on their way to the airport that he found out what was going on. They arrived just in time for Gamila to make her flight.

She paused and took a deep breath before she maneuvered out of the truck. Pregnancy has a tendency to slow you down. Gamila was moving as fast as her body would allow.

Chapter Twelve

Discipline/Alternatives

Once Gamila started treating Chris at home his overall condition improved. She knew then that it was time to be a little more aggressive in disciplining him. But how do you discipline a child with a bleeding disorder?

Gamila remembered her aunt disciplining her cousins when they were young. Her aunt would make the boys do push-ups, or stand in a corner holding books and counting for thirty minutes to an hour, or they had to write down whatever it was they weren't supposed to do again—five hundred times.

The problem was that it just wasn't possible to use any of those methods with Chris. He'd be able to do the push-ups, but not enough to be considered a punishment without causing a bleed. Standing for a long period of time while holding books would put pressure on his knees, ankles, and heels, so that idea was scratched off the list. Writing a sentence five hundred times could give him a bleed in his hand because of the repetitive motion. Chris did play a lot of video games, but only in short intervals. Gamila considered the writing punishment, but the whole idea was to make the child do it in one sitting and that just wasn't possible without causing a bleed.

Gamila was lucky in that she didn't need to punish Chris often, but all kids have their moments, and she had to find something she could do. Since Chris loved video games so much, Gamila had to resort to taking away his games for a week or so as punishment. This worked well when he was young, but as he got older it was no longer enough.

Chris was always a nice, respectful child—and now he's a nice, respectful young man. But no matter what Gamila tried, she always had a difficult time getting him to clean. He absolutely hated cleaning.

Gamila thinks that being immobilized so often, and spending so much time in a hospital during his first few years, explains why it was hard to get Chris to cooperate in this. When children are toddlers they're usually starting to learn to put away their toys. But because Chris was in a hospital bed, or having to stay still while his body healed from a bleed, everyone else was picking up after him. Gamila felt that all this contributed to making Chris a little lazy when it came to cleaning up after himself.

She was sensitive to his circumstances, but she was still a parent. When Chris was little she was able to explain the importance of cleanliness and moving his body. Eventually, she got him to the point of actually picking up his toys and putting things away, even at The Hospital.

Things weren't so easy once he became an adolescent and Gamila expected him to do more chores. He utterly cringed at the idea of sweeping or mopping a floor. And forget about asking him to do the dishes, that almost brought tears to his eyes. Gamila explained that it wasn't fair to his sister if he didn't have to clean too, and he would eventually do what he was told, but it took him forever.

Chris understood that he had to have chores just as his sister did, but the issue still remained something of a problem. Gamila was grateful that cleaning was her only real issue with Chris, but for her, it wasn't simply about his chores. She was worried about him developing poor habits. She was afraid that his lackadaisical attitude to doing what he was supposed to do would get out of control as he got older, and she didn't want Chris's attitude to give him another handicap.

"If you get in the habit of putting things off until tomorrow, there will come a time when you'll realize that you should have done it today," she tried to explain. But it just wasn't working.

Gamila had to find a way to change his behavior. She discussed the issue with her sister. Gamila's sister suggested adding a task to Chris's usual punishment and Gamila thought it was a great idea. Whenever Chris had to be told more than twice to do his chores he was put on punishment.

Chris's aunt gave him guidelines for writing book reports. She also gave him a desktop computer and showed him how to use Microsoft Word. When he got in trouble with his mom he had to read a book of his choice and write a book report. His aunt set the due date for the report. She would critique and grade it, and if it needed any changes she handed it back to him for corrections. Chris wasn't allowed to play at all—and he certainly couldn't play video games—until the report was finished to his aunt's satisfaction.

Turns out, Chris ended up liking the book reports and he became an excellent writer and communicator. Once he reached high school he made the debate team and they won several state and local competitions. Chris won a college scholarship in one of his last debates. It goes without saying that Gamila was extremely proud of her son.

A Sample of Chris's Winning Debate (age 16):

"When I was a kid, I used to play in the biggest box I could find. I would imagine I was a king ruling my cardboard kingdom. As most kids do, I oozed innocence and was a king determined to rule my domain with tranquility and kindness. From Teddy Bear Tower to Candy Cane Lane my kingdom would be the best in the world. But as we grow older our childhood and important things we learned during these carefree days seem to take a backseat. Things like "treat others the way you want to be treated" become just a phrase and when you try to look for the best in the darkest of people you're deemed naive as if those shadowy living creatures are incapable of kindness. But the child in me that's lived freely for years now lives in fear of what I've become. When did I become so mean? Maybe in 2009 when it was reported that a person took their own life every 14.2 minutes or perhaps when it was reported over 77% of students experienced bullying regularly. These statistics aren't just numbers but loved ones we've all lost. Mothers, fathers, children, and friends, we're all fighting our own battles.

Although we can't predict everything life throws at us, we can control how to react. When we take the risk of trusting someone, we wrap our heart in a box, and gently scribble handle with care on the side. So when someone entrust me with this delicate package, I know I can't treat it like another piece of junk mail that I throw on the counter as I return home. The child inside me hides behind this shell of maturity but he burns through brighter than any sunlight ever could when this package is put at risk. So this is why I stand in front of you today. To figure out why are we so mean to each other? To solve the problem, we must first ask and answer 3 questions.

- What makes people in today's society so cold?
- Can we avoid being hurt in today's cruel society?
- How can we make a change?

My 1st area of analysis: Merriam Webster dictionary conveys being cold as depressing and gloomy.

So the strong negativity in today's society says more about how people feel about themselves than how they feel about you. Considering Nathan Heflick of Psychology Today, states "When our self-esteem is threatened, we are more likely to compare ourselves to people we think are worse off than us." So the root of everyone else's insecurities are our own. Those who feel lost seek comfort and strength any way they can find it. People make more of an impact than words can ever say when joined together. However, when we let hatred corrupt us and we join together to hurt others it leads to nothing but complete chaos. When negativity infects us we turn from a group of civil disobedience to an angry riot force.

But misery loves company and it feels good to be accepted into a group so we let our own insecurities affect the way we treat others. So stand tall and allow your confidence to be contagious, become the turning point in someone else's life.

There are limitless variables that shape a person's character from the people in their life to the situations that happened to them. These variables mold our desire for power, comfort, security, attention, and other cravings we may have. Children that are neglected by parents often go into an attention seeking state which makes children search for attention by ways of bullying and self-harm. Children with parents who work long hours and are rarely seen, children who grew up in a broken household missing mothers or fathers. Even people that appear even-keel can show signs of feeling neglected.

My 2nd area of Analysis: Those of us who decide to be disrespectful are causing an emotional domino effect that passes from person to person knocking down our confidence in hopes to take attention off themselves. So to stop the domino effect we have to be stronger than the rest. Unfortunately, not every kid was taught how to be strong and persevere, so those who stand up for the girl who's slightly bigger than the rest, those who do good and expect nothing in return, and those who are careful to hear the claims and opinions of others but not let them shape their reality so they can better themselves as a person, knows what being strong means. My mother, a black woman who singlehandedly raised 4 kids showed the little boy in his cardboard castle what it took to be strong every day of her life. She showed him that to support a family you had to wake up every day at 5:00 A.M. to get the kids ready for school. Have breakfast on the table by 6:25 so you can be ready for work by 6:55. Leave the house by 7:30, get to work by 8:00, work until 3:00 only to pick up the kids at 3:30. Get home at 6:00 so you can finish dinner by 7:00. Help the kids with their homework at 8:00 then have the house clean by 9:00 and be up on time the next morning like clockwork and she never missed a step. She showed him the things a father behind bars wasn't able to – how to tie a tie and how to change a tire and how to treat a lady. She showed him that no matter how hard you bust your butt to be the best you can be, there will always be someone who doesn't approve and that's just the way the world works. So I learned a long time ago what it took to be strong and I would make sure that strength my mother passed to me would continue to be passed on.

I know, it almost sounds as if I was suggesting that we lay our weapons down and live in a fictional existence of happily ever after, but, allow me to clarify. I'm suggesting we learn to take better control over our emotions and not allow our emotions to take control of us. Scott Adams, creator of the Dilbert comic stirp, once said "Nothing defines humans better than their willingness to do irrational things in the pursuit of phenomenally unlikely payoffs." The truth is, we as humans have an uncanny ability to act irrationally or to not act at all, but the challenge is finding the balance. If we take the time to think before allowing our emotions to rule and practice empathy for others then maybe we won't have to constantly have to fight for happiness, we can just allow it to happen. As long as we maintain patience and diligence we can change the world, one person at a time. Can one person really change the world? How much of a difference can one person make? Maybe we can ask Martin Luther King Jr. or Elizabeth Stanton if one person can change the world. The point is there is nothing in the world we as people can't do. From space exploration to exploring the depths of the ocean we've done so much and to tell the truth we've only scratched the surface. The only thing standing in our way is ourselves. Are we ready to make the change?

My 3rd area of analysis: In order to make the change we have to renew some of the older principles we teach our kids but refuse to use ourselves. Treat others the way you want to be treated, no one wants to feel hurt so why do people go out of their way to intentionally hurt others. If you have nothing nice to say don't say anything at all. Whether in real life or on social media, spiteful comments have indirectly snatched the lives of those we love away from us. Most importantly, we don't always hurt others on purpose so when we do hurt others, a simple, "I'm sorry" is the least we can do.

I realized a long time ago I wasn't really a king. I realized that my cardboard castle was nothing more than a box that had handle with care gently scribbled on the side. I realized that my residents were nothing more than superman action figures and toy dogs with ripped collars. However, one thing remained constant, the child that lived in that cardboard castle is still there. So whenever I'm going astray that kid pulls me back in, he pulls me back to my senses and I remember, I remember when I used to be a king, I remember how things used to be. The child in all of us knows what's right so just because our childhood is over doesn't mean we should keep them locked away. Let them run free in their own cardboard kingdom and usher in an era of prosperity."

* * *

Chris had to grow up strong and fast. He wasn't a typical toddler, adolescent, or teenager. This was both a blessing and a curse. His natural intelligence allowed him to gain insights into life at a young age, but his condition prevented him from doing normal childhood activities.

Spending so much time at The Hospital as a baby and toddler taught him to understand his condition, and how to manage it. He learned early on that his physical disability didn't have to determine the direction of his life. He came to accept the things he wouldn't be able to do and to capitalize on the things he was comfortable doing. He learned to alter his direction to fit his life.

Chris is a calm, charismatic, and respectful young man. He never gave Gamila any real trouble. And with the help of her sister's book report punishments, Gamila prevented him from gaining an attitude problem.

Even though Chris's life has been painful, he hasn't allowed that to poison his mind with bitterness and hard feelings. He has integrity, he's sensitive to the suffering and needs of others, and he has a deep appreciation for life.

Of course, Chris wasn't always this way. His mindset took years to develop as he adapted to his condition and learned not to let it hold him back. But all in all, he was a good kid growing up, and he's turned into a wonderful young man.

Chapter Thirteen

Steel-Toe Boots

In 2006 Gamila found out she was pregnant with her third child. With a small waist, flat tummy, broad hips, and a dream butt, Gamila's body was desired by most men and envied by many women. But when it came to pregnancy, Gamila's bodacious body caused her some trouble.

Her unborn baby never wanted to ride up front. The child always seemed to want to be along her lower back, lingering near her side in a neat little ball as if it was afraid of exposing itself to the world. This preference of her unborn made it almost impossible to tell that Gamila was pregnant, and it made it difficult for doctors to determine how far along she was.

This peculiar positioning also ensured that Gamila endured a lot of pain during pregnancy, because the baby weighed her down and put additional pressure on her hips. But it wasn't until this pregnancy that Gamila was finally referred to a chiropractor.

The first time she walked into the chiropractor's office she was hunched over in pain, inching along at turtle speed. The office assistants thought she didn't look pregnant at all.

After about thirty minutes of a twist here and a turn there, Gamila was good as new. The pain was gone and she could walk upright. The office assistants were amazed when they saw her after the treatment. They could definitely tell that she was pregnant now.

Chiropractic treatments would be frequent during this pregnancy, along with visits to other doctors that weren't nearly as satisfying. Whenever Gamila got pregnant she had to attend "counseling consultation sessions" so the doctors could "go over your options." They maintained, "It's in your best interest." They also made it clear that refusing to attend the sessions would be considered medical neglect.

* * *

It was a bitter cold day, although warmer than one would expect for Michigan in January. The sun's rays soothingly glazed the perfect blanket of snow that covered the grass.

Gamila's third pregnancy was difficult. She'd been sick throughout most of it, and so had Al.

As she walked to the truck that morning she remembered one time they were doing seventy miles an hour when all of a sudden Al swerved over to the right shoulder of the road and slammed on the brakes. She was confused and started hurling questions at him but he didn't answer. It was only after he bolted out of the truck and ran over to the passenger side to eject the contents of his gut that she understood.

The whole thing was scary, and quite disturbing, but once Gamila understood what was going on—and confirmed that he was OK—she couldn't help but smirk. Women have wanted men to feel the pain and challenges of pregnancy since the dawn of time. That was one of those times. As far as Gamila was concerned, it was perfect.

She had mixed emotions as she started the truck and headed off to her next appointment. Pregnant women expect to have many doctor's visits, but Gamila had to endure more than most. Not to mention, some of the visits seemed like a total waste of time and nothing more than a chance for the doctor to do unnecessary probing of her and her unborn child. If the baby was a boy there'd be further tests and probing, but she was excited to find out the child's sex nonetheless.

Mount Clemens had the feel of a small, old-fashioned town. In fact, it almost seemed uninhabited. Just before 8 a.m., Gamila turned onto a side street. The dusting of snow on the deserted street was undisturbed, but smog seemed to have replaced the air. This haze had become typical for southern Michigan. The people who lived in the area were used to *pollution shock*.

Gamila scanned her surroundings. The street was lined with traditional small town buildings and black streetlamps that hugged the curbs. There were only a few cars in the diagonal parking spaces in front of the buildings.

"Am I in the right place? Where are the addresses? I know it has to be over here somewhere, but how am I supposed to know which building it is?" She wanted to turn around and head back home, but she kept moving.

It wasn't until she saw something familiar—a UPS truck—that she decided she was in the right place. "All right, I guess this is it. . . finally," she said with as much excitement as she could muster given that the cold gloom had begun weighing on her. "I don't wanna park too far and have to walk a long way." She gently tapped her fingers on the top of the steering wheel before pulling into one of the empty spaces and turning off the ignition. "Pregnancy is definitely something to be *desired*," she announced with a long sigh as she scooted out of the truck.

Gamila walked to the front door of the medical office. The small window in the middle of the worn door was covered by a note with an arrow directing people to a rear entrance.

She walked to the end of the formidable row of small businesses, around a corner, and into a creepy alleyway. *I'm sure this can't be the way in. This looks like some kind of freaky Friday the 13th movie.* "Where's Jason?" she muttered just as she noticed the UPS man entering the building. *This must be the way.*

An enormous dumpster partially blocked the path to the back entrance of the office. An anxious feeling knotted Gamila's stomach, but she wasn't going to be deterred from the task at hand.

What she wasn't ready to do was explore her "other options"—or endure their "recommended precautions"—before she knew what she was up against. Doctors had already advised her to take an amniocentesis[9] test to find out if her unborn baby had any birth defects. "Why put the baby and me under more stress if it may not be needed?" she'd asked

---

[9] Amniocentesis is a prenatal test in which a small amount of amniotic fluid is removed from the sac surrounding the fetus for testing. It is performed to look for certain types of birth defects. Source: www.webmd.com/baby/guide/amniocentesis

them. The doctors had also been trying to sway her to terminate the pregnancy. Gamila was familiar with some of their scheming strategies because they'd used the same tactics when she was pregnant with her second child.

Gamila stepped inside the office. The place appeared empty. There was no sign of life at all—no receptionist, no kids, no one. Where is everybody? she thought.

Any remaining hopeful thoughts about this should-be-beautiful occasion evaporated when a pair of steel-toe boots came into focus. Gamila assumed the woman in army fatigue pants was a nurse.

Unnerving thoughts flooded Gamila's mind like arsenic flowing through a bloodstream as she followed the woman through the open double doors and into the examination room. What the hell? What is this lady wearing? She looks like a serial killer, thought Gamila. She was baffled by the woman's bizarre appearance, to say the least.

Her unease intensified when she learned that the steel-toe boot lady was the doctor. Since when do doctors come to the waiting room themselves to get their patients? wondered Gamila.

The doctor left her alone in the examination room to get changed. She felt she needed to be prepared for the unexpected, especially since all the doctors and nurses had been insisting that she have the amniocentesis test or consider terminating the pregnancy.

After undressing and putting on the tissue examination gown Gamila scouted the room for a weapon, just in case. She quietly opened drawers in search of something she could use for protection. She found a surgical needle, unwrapped it, and slid the needle under the paper cover as she sat on the exam table.

"Are you nervous?" the doctor asked as she entered the room. "Don't be. This ultrasound will be a cinch for you. You've already had two children, right?"

"Yes," said Gamila. She was nervous, but about the doctor—not the ultrasound.

"All right then, let's get started." The doctor smiled as she disconcertingly pulled the edge of one of her latex gloves and let it go, snapping it against her wrist.

This freaky Jason lady is a weirdo, thought Gamila. I'm glad I have that needle. . . this is a trip.

The doctor confirmed that Gamila's unborn baby was male. She wasn't surprised. She'd suspected all along that she was carrying a boy.

* * *

After Gamila found out she was having a baby boy the doctors began hounding her to have the amniocentesis test to determine if her unborn son had any birth defects. Gamila wasn't going to make a decision until she weighed her options and did a little research.

She learned that the amniocentesis test could cause a miscarriage, bleeding, leaking of amniotic fluid,[10] an infection, or possible preterm labor. She was misdiagnosed with Chris, and the doctors' probing may have caused some of his illnesses. She didn't want to take that chance with this baby. Furthermore, no doctor ever concretely established that she was a carrier of the hemophilia gene. Gamila had a feeling she was a carrier, but the doctors weren't able to determine this. She decided the test wasn't an option for her.

The doctors were not pleased with her decision. They tried to insist she have the test. "If you have the test and the results are positive, you can consider terminating the pregnancy. It can be terminated up to twenty-seven weeks," said one doctor.

That's preposterous, she thought. It's a full-grown baby at twenty-seven weeks.

---

[10] The amniotic fluid is like the water in a pregnant woman. It's a clear yellowish liquid surrounding the fetus in the amniotic sac during pregnancy.
Source: www.nlm.nih.gov/medlineplus/ency/article/002220.htm

Doctor after doctor shamelessly revealed the real reason they were trying to push her into terminating the pregnancy. "You should strongly consider having an abortion. . . it would be better for the economy. If you have another child with hemophilia there will be a lot of costs involved and it will negatively impact the health care industry," another doctor explained.

Gamila couldn't believe what she was hearing—again. She'd already endured over twenty months of nagging and probing through all her pregnancies. She'd reached her limit. The doctors didn't count on the fact that Gamila could be just as frank as they were. After listening tirelessly to doctor after doctor explain the importance of this "termination" decision, she was going to speak her mind.

Gamila's nostrils flared. She stared the doctor straight in the eye, rocked her head, and said, "Please stop acting like you care about my well-being. Dr. Felts already explained that if this baby is born with hemophilia it would be costly to the *government*, or *health insurance companies*, or *whoever*. I really don't give a damn about all that. My primary concern is for the welfare of my child, caring for my other children, and my family. So you can stop with the nonsense because terminating my pregnancy is *not* an option, and if you ask me again it's going to be a problem."

That shut this particular doctor up, but it wasn't the end of it. Gamila had no choice but to continue attending these "counseling consultation sessions." The doctors were trying to wear her down. They wanted to convince her that their way was the only way.

Regardless of how frustrating it was, and no matter how crude the doctors' tactics, she couldn't even tell Al what was going on. He would've been pissed and never would've trusted another doctor again.

* * *

Gamila and Al were worn out from all her visits to doctors. Many of the visits were completely unnecessary and they were taking their toll. The couple were exasperated.

They'd overslept this morning. Now they were running late for her next "counseling consultation session."

"You got everything you need babe?" asked Al, trying to focus his sleepy eyes.

"Yeah, I got everything," said Gamila as she yawned. She was moving as quickly as she could. "But I already told you I don't want to go. I know what this is about and I don't want to hear it. I'm tired and in pain right now."

"I know babe, but it's going to be OK."

Gamila's real reason for not wanting to go escaped Al, but she knew it was better that way. All he knew was that she had a doctor's appointment and he needed to get her there on time. He never gave it much thought beyond that. Al didn't want her to have to drive anywhere by herself, and he always insisted on taking her if he could. He was like that. If he had his way she wouldn't ever have had to drive anywhere alone.

Al's snow driving skills were superb. They arrived at the doctor's office with a couple of minutes to spare.

"You and my sister can get anybody where they need to go, *on time*, no matter what," Gamila said with a faint laugh.

He laughed. "I just didn't want you to be late babe. I'm sorry I overslept. Are you OK? You still in pain?"

"I'll be fine. Let's just get this over with."

Gamila wished she didn't have to continue entertaining these doctors. Maybe one day one of them will say something useful, she thought. But I'm not holding my breath.

Her name was called before she and Al had a chance to sit down. They were directed to examination room three.

Gamila made a beeline for the cozy-looking chair stationed in the corner. She flopped down and relaxed her lower back on the lumbar support. Her elbow dug into the arm and she rested her forehead against her unclenched fist. Al sat on the examination table, as if he was the patient. They were having a quiet laugh that came to a halt when the doctor knocked on the door.

The doctor entered the room with a bright smile. "How are mom and baby doing?" he pleasantly asked.

"Fine," said Gamila. She knew the real reason for this visit. She couldn't stop thinking about the doctor's ill intentions, and she wasn't going to give him any extra information—any extra ammunition—if she could help it.

The doctor went on about how beautiful pregnancy is, how wonderful life is, and how grand the world is. He completely failed to capture Gamila's interest with his tall tales of pregnancy bliss. In fact, she was practically zoning him out.

Al, however, was listening with great interest. He was hanging on the doctor's every word, but he soon interrupted the happy little speech. "So, doc, what exactly is the purpose of this visit?"

"Well," said the doctor, "we know how hard this decision can be for a couple, and we want you to know that it's one that many couples have made in the past. We just want what's best for mom and the baby."

"Doc, you're dancing around something and I'm not sure what it is. You need to just spit it out," Al insisted.

The doctor looked over at Gamila. "Have you given any thought to terminating the pregnancy?"

"What?" Al's eyes got huge and his strong voice got even deeper. "*What* did you just ask her?"

The doctor turned to face Gamila. "Well, given the circumstances with your first child, you know, having hemophilia A, we just thought it would be something you would consider. . . since it has been confirmed that the unborn baby you're carrying is a boy."

Gamila said nothing. She just wanted to go home and lie down. If she had a choice she wouldn't attend any of these "counseling consultation sessions." She rested her cheek on her hand and waited for Al to deliver his wrath.

"Have you lost your damn mind man?" The question was rhetorical. Al didn't wait for an answer. "You must be crazy as hell! You're asking her to KILL MY BABY? You're out of your mind!" Al was practically frothing at the mouth. He stood up, his six-foot-seven frame towering over the doctor.

"No . . . no, we're simply letting her know her options," the doctor backtracked. He'd been nice and calm up to that point, but Al clearly made him nervous. "It is ultimately your decision," the doctor said to Gamila.

"Let's get out of here babe. I've heard enough." Al helped Gamila out of the chair.

The doctor focused on Gamila again. "It's ultimately your decision, and it is something to consider, given the circumstances. The cost of the termination would be covered, and you could go on to provide complete care to your firstborn with hemophilia. This bleeding disorder is typically passed down through the mother, and you could be a carrier of the gene. Your unborn could suffer with this as well."

"Look you cocksucker, she is NOT killing my baby, plain and simple," said Al with even more conviction.

You keep saying that the cost of an abortion would be covered, but how about you provide some support and help me with the costs of caring for Chris? thought Gamila. How about that?

She'd encountered nothing but problem after problem while caring for Chris. The only thing this doctor's visit achieved was dredging up bad memories of all the frustrations and challenges she'd faced—and overcome—while caring for her firstborn.

Gamila was frankly sick and tired of the doctors talking about a termination. There was a life inside her and she wasn't going to let the doctors dictate her baby's course. She'd never even considered having an abortion. It simply was not an option. She had, of course, given some thought to this baby being born with a bleeding disorder, but the only thing she could do was cross that bridge if and when she reached it.

Al and Gamila left the doctor's office. Neither of them felt much like talking. The drive home was pretty quiet.

*   *   *

Doctors were ready for a better delivery this time, precautions were taken. They used special tools to pull the baby out just in case he had a bleeding disorder.

Julian was born big and healthy. The doctors performed several tests and it was determined that he didn't have hemophilia. That was a relief for Gamila.

Chris was nine when Julian was born. He asked if his brother had the same condition he did.

"Well, the doctors ran some tests and he doesn't have a bleeding disorder," Gamila answered.

"Why doesn't he have hemophilia?" Chris seemed sort of upset. "I mean. . . I'm happy Julian doesn't have hemophilia, but it makes me wonder why I have it. Why did this only happen to me?"

"I know baby. Some things just happen to people for reasons unknown. That's a part of life and there's nothing we can do about that. But we'll get through this. We will not let it dictate our path. You understand?"

"Yeah, I do. I'm happy my brother doesn't have this mess." Chris smiled. "I wouldn't want him to go through what I've been through."

"I know," said Gamila. "And just think, you get to teach him everything you know." She was trying to make Chris excited about having a baby brother.

A wide smile spread across Chris's face. "Yeah, you're right."

One day Chris mentioned to his mother that he wished there was a cure for hemophilia so he could live a better life and not have to worry about taking his medication or being injured just from walking up and down a flight of stairs. But as he grew up he came to terms with his condition and learned to make the most of his life.

* * *

Gamila's healthy baby boy, Julian. Julian in a *Minute to Win It* contest at school as he tries to balance blocks on a paper plate on top of his head.

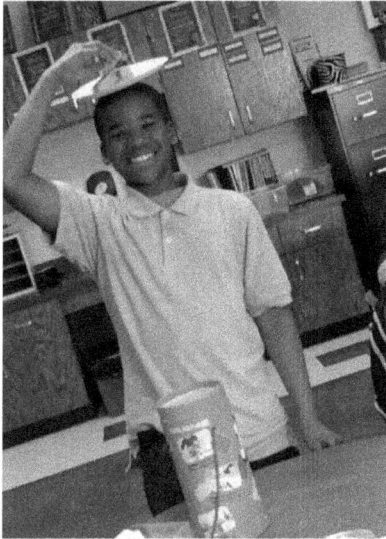

He's handsome, bright and in a gifted class in school. Julian loves to play basketball and was on a little league flag football team. He loves to draw and is pretty good at it. He wants to be an architect.

Gamila was disappointed when the doctors tried to convince her that it would be in the *best interest of the child* to terminate the pregnancy. "Life is life, you never know what hand you will be dealt...you just have to learn to work with what you have and be able to quickly adjust along the way," Gamila would say.

Chapter Fourteen

This is Our Life!

Jaden was born in 2008. During her pregnancy, Gamila somehow felt he would be a boy with hemophilia. She couldn't explain how she knew, but she knew.

Jaden's blood tests came back positive. It was heart-wrenching for Gamila to think about watching another child go through the pain and agony that Chris had gone through—that he will go through forever. But Jaden is smart, vivacious, and clever, and Gamila wouldn't trade him for the world.

Gamila knew she was in for another challenge, but she was better-prepared this time. She had a doctor who cared and an excellent hematology clinic for the boys' routine appointments and comprehensive clinical visits. Gamila can't imagine where she would be today without the support of her family—and the right doctor who cares about Chris's and Jaden's well-being.

Chris has chronic pain and limited mobility due to soft tissue and bone damage to his knee from years of repeated hemorrhages. Jaden is learning to deal with his condition under the guidance of his brother.

Chris recently had to see an orthopedic surgeon about his knee. He was told he has osteoarthritis and the surgeon has recommended knee replacement surgery within the next few months. Chris and Gamila are preparing for another uphill battle, but they have strong hope that the surgery will improve his mobility and reduce his pain.

Somehow, through all the hospital stays, treatments, and scare tactics, Gamila and her children are still standing tall. As the boys and their mother continue to work through difficult times, what Gamila does know is that they are determined to make it!

* * *

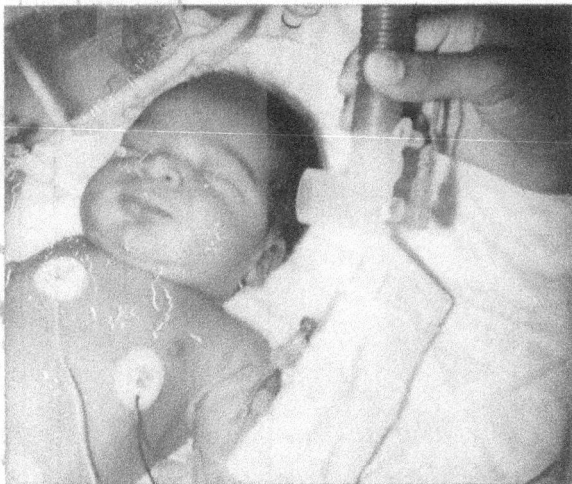

Newborn Chris in the hospital. (above)

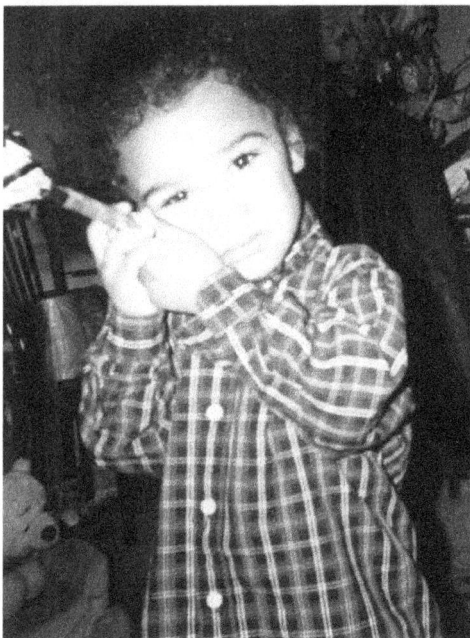

Little Chris age 2.

Chris, in the hospital. (below) Gamila had to post notes all over his bed because nurses were trying to draw blood by poking his fingers instead of going through the IV. Hospital staff frequently forgot to pull the bed rails back up. These are things that the staff should have been conscious about, especially for a four-year-old with a bleeding disorder, but unfortunately, none of these "typical" procedures were followed by all.

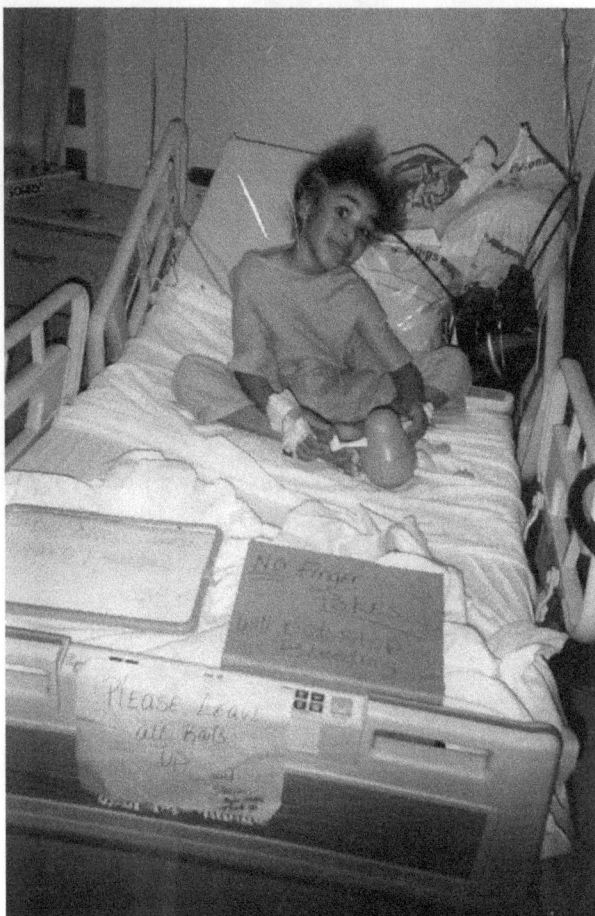

Chris at Disney World.

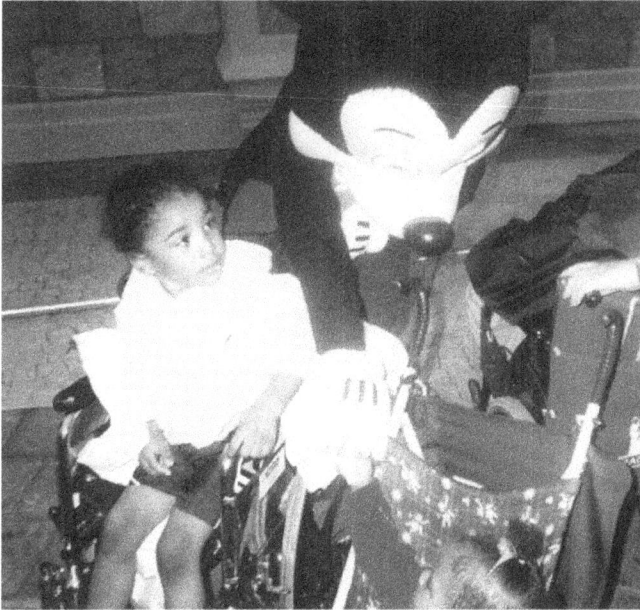

A family trip courtesy of Make-a-Wish foundation. Chris (above) meeting Mickey Mouse. Chris (below) appreciating his gifts from Mickey, Goofy, and Minnie!

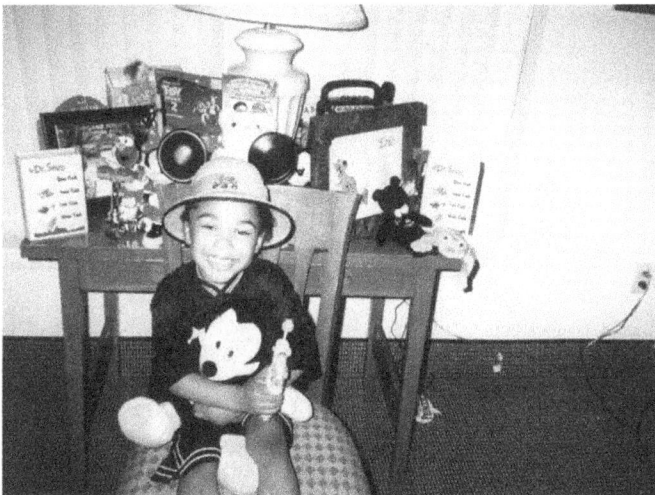

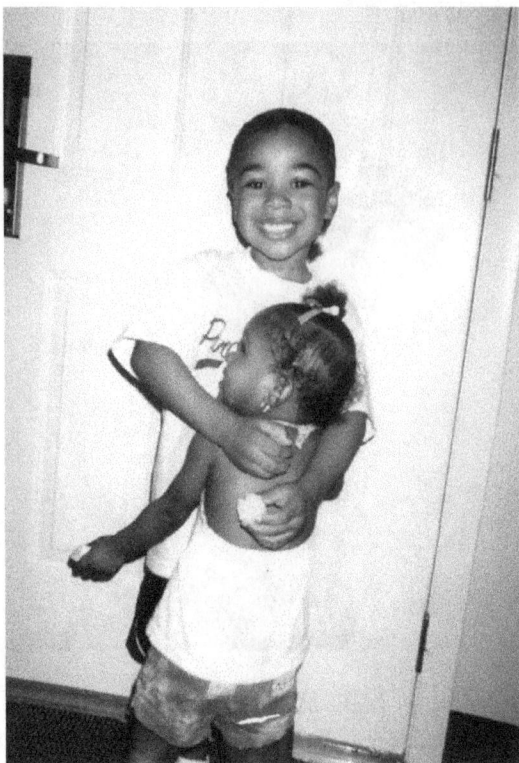

Chris with his little sister, Azha. Chris, age 4 and Azha, age 2. (left)

Chris after one of his visits to the hematology clinic. (below)

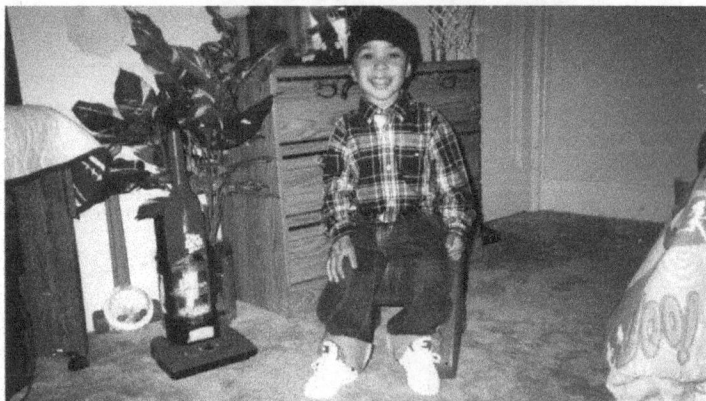

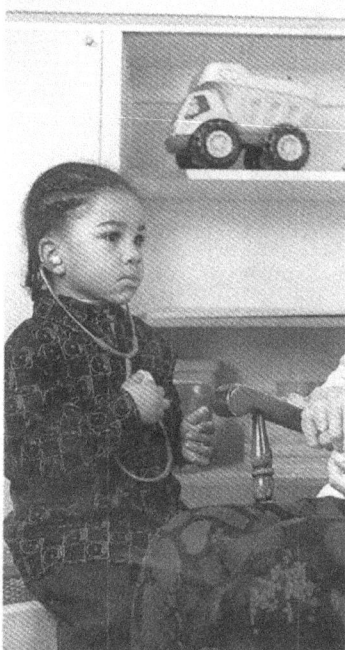

Chris in a University article that featured one of The Hospital's Hematology specialist discussing Gene Therapy. (left)

ems
plus
) be
the
Dr.
d.
that
ls is
nder
cau-
atch-
the
)rug
)n's
rapy
ier's
e, is
dard
pro-
first
trial
)wer
.iral

Chris, a proud big brother, pushing his little sister on the swings at the playground.

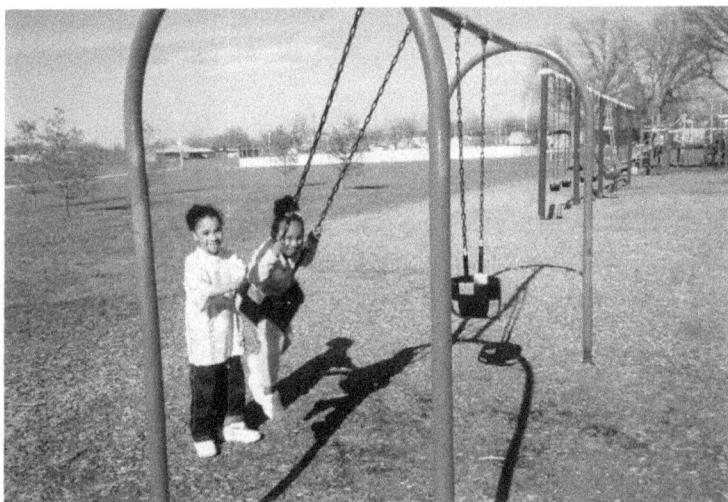

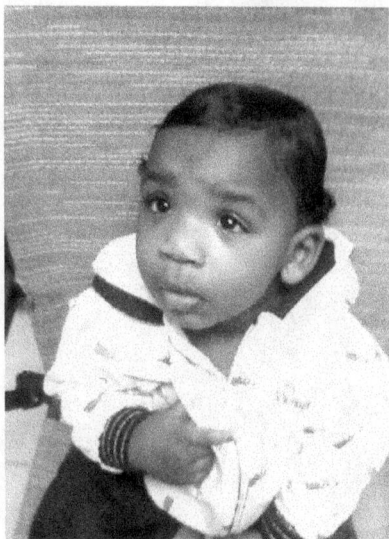

Jaden (left) eight months old. Also diagnosed with Severe Hemophilia A at birth.

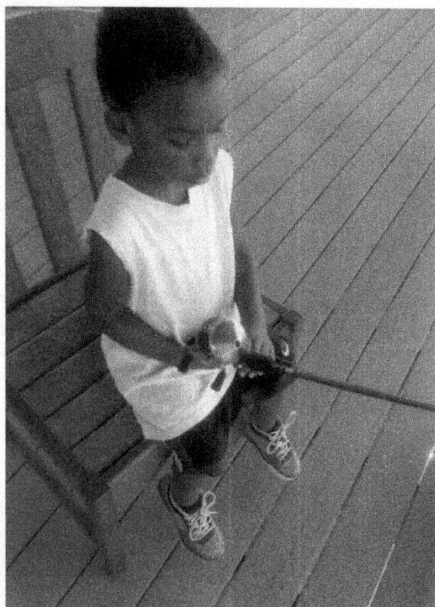

Jaden (right) age 3. Enjoying himself as he learns to fish at a hemophilia camp.

Hemophilia History

Hemophilia has been part of recorded history since the second century. There are reports of male babies dying after circumcision and young males bleeding to death from minor injuries. However, the name hemophilia wasn't given to the disease until the 1800s. Generally speaking, females are the carriers of the gene while the disease manifests mostly in males.

Hemophilia became known as the royal disease when it was discovered that Queen Victoria of England was a carrier of the gene. According to the British Medical Journal, Leopold, her eighth child, had hemophilia. He had frequent blood hemorrhages and he eventually died of a brain bleed at age thirty-one. Leopold passed the gene to his daughter Alice who was a carrier. She passed the disease to her son Viscount Trematon, and he died of a brain hemorrhage in 1928. The disease affected German, Russian, and Spanish royal families, and the carriers were all descended from Queen Victoria.

The royals resorted to hypnosis and other unconventional ways of controlling bleeds. Most notably, Tsarina Alexandra of Russia fell under the influence of the infamous monk Rasputin because he was somehow able to control the bleeding of her hemophiliac son Alexei.

Doctors were able to offer better treatment options by the mid-twentieth century. It was determined that a protein in the blood could help the clotting factors of an individual with hemophilia, and doctors began using fresh blood plasma to treat bleeding episodes. Unfortunately, using whole blood still left the majority of the individuals who suffered from a bleeding disorder crippled, and they usually died from repeated hemorrhages. Tragedy struck when over half the individuals with hemophilia in the US contracted HIV and Hepatitis-C from contaminated blood.

Testing and research continued, leading to new developments and safer treatment methods. Individuals who suffer from a bleeding disorder today have access to antihemophilic factor (recombinant) plasma products. An antihemophilic factor (recombinant) is a glycoprotein synthesized product used to treat bleeding episodes in individuals with a factor VIII deficiency, and it is also used for the prevention and control of hemorrhagic episodes.[11]

---

[11] Source:
www.fda.gov/BiologicsBloodVaccines/BloodBloodProducts/Approve
dProducts/LicensedProductsBLAs/FractionatedPlasmaProducts/ucm
200417.htm

Xyntha Solofuse—brand name Advate—is the factor VIII replacement therapy medication used by Chris and Jaden.

According to the Canadian Hemophilia Society,[12] about twenty-five percent of individuals diagnosed with hemophilia don't receive the proper care they need to live long, productive lives. A person with hemophilia lives a life of pain, and without the proper treatment they can suffer even more pain, crippling, and die an early death.

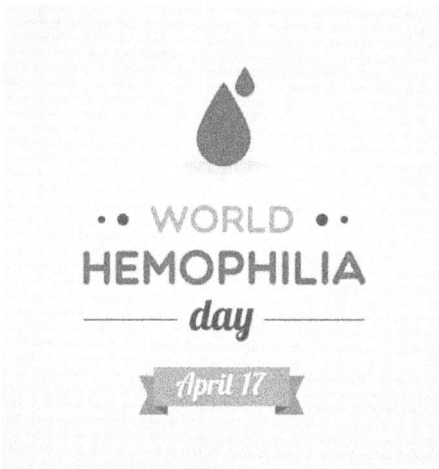

---

[12]Canadian Hemophilia Society, The history of hemophilia, http://www.hemophilia.ca/bleeding-disorders

Acknowledgement

This would come to be one of my most challenging books that I've ever written. My sister, Eric and Jaden were the biggest inspiration for writing this book. Even though *Through the Eyes of a Mother* would be the most difficult to write, it would also be the most *rewarding*. It is not difficult, however, to express my deepest thanks to my sister who allowed me to write her story. I just hope I conveyed the story as she would have wanted it told! A special thank you to my sister's Home Care Consultants, Carletha and Harvey Gates for going above and beyond to ensure that my nephew had the medication and supplies he needed when he needed it; as well as keeping us informed of national hemophilia conferences, camps, and the like. Thank you Carletha. Last but certainly not least, I would like to thank my family for supporting me in all my writing endeavors.

Appendix
Helpful Resources

These resources have been gathered and provided to you as a starting point. They are by no means the only sources available, and they should not be taken as the *only* solution or place to find what you may be searching for. We've done some extensive research to generate this list but please keep in mind that businesses move, phone numbers change, and many businesses are combining companies and resources. And remember, never be afraid to ask questions – the life of your child depends on you!

Organizations/Associations

- National Hemophilia Association, New York, NY (800) 424-2634, www.hemophilia.org

- Hemophilia Federation of America, Washington, DC – (202) 675-6984, www.hemophiliafed.org

- National Organization for Rare Disorders
  (NORD) - www.rarediseases.org

- World Federation of Hemophilia
  https://www.wfh.org

Assistance Programs

- Helping Hands, www.hemophiliafed.org
- Patient Assistance Programs - HemAware
  www.hemaware.org

Or, search for "Hemophilia Help" and put the <u>state</u> you live in to generate a list of places that provide assistance for families who have children that suffer from a bleeding disorder.

Bad Blood: A Cautionary Tale, Directed by Marilyn Ness. To learn more about the contaminated blood, view the 2010 documentary. Visit the app **IMDb** or stream from **Amazon.com.**

About the Author

Alina has written the internationally sold debut novel "Deceptive Men" and the methodical twisted tale "Mrs. Deveraux". This is Alina's first non-fiction book, "Through the Eyes of a Mother". Alina still currently works in her lifelong field of accounting and finance – holding a degree in accounting and worked for several Fortune 100 companies. She lives in Texas with her family. For more updated information, visit www.alinabooks.com.

www.ingramcontent.com/pod-product-compliance
Lightning Source LLC
Chambersburg PA
CBHW071054040426
42443CB00013B/3330